HOW TO LOWER YOUR FAT THERMOSTAT

The No-Diet Reprogramming Plan for
Lifelong Weight Control

HOW TO LOWER YOUR FAT THERMOSTAT

The No-Diet Reprogramming Plan for
Lifelong Weight Control

Dennis W. Remington, M.D.
A. Garth Fisher, Ph.D.
Edward A. Parent, Ph.D.

Vitality House International, Inc.

Copyright 1983 by
Vitality House International, Inc.
1675 North Freedom Blvd. #11-C
Provo, Utah 84604

Telephone: 801-373-5100
To Order: Call Toll Free 1-800-637-0708

First Printing, April 1983
Second Printing, June 1983
Third Printing, November 1983
Fourth Printing, June 1984
Fifth Printing, April 1985
Sixth Printing, January 1986
Seventh Printing, March 1987
Eighth Printing, December 1987
Ninth Printing, March 1988
Tenth Printing, October 1988
Eleventh Printing, June 1989
Twelfth Printing, April 1990

Library of Congress Catalog Card Number: 83-80794

ISBN 0-912547-01-4

Printed in the United States of America

Table of Contents

Appendices

List of Diagrams

List of Tables

Preface

The authors first associated together in early 1981 bringing a broad experience in exercise physiology, medicine, and psychology into a comprehensive weight-management program. Although we were realizing modest success (comparable to any other multi-modal approaches) we were not satisfied with our results.

We had all been reading the literature relating to weight management and were excited when we read the new ideas concerning the weight-regulating mechanism, setpoint, and energy conservation and wasting. As we continued our study, it became clear that the conventional approaches to weight control would never work and we began to develop treatment principles to lower the setpoint so that the body would allow excess fat to be lost naturally and permanently.

Our first attempts to lower the setpoint were rewarding and many of our patients responded beautifully. However, at the time we still restricted the intake of food to less than 1,000 calories a day for patients who had a serious problem and some of them made little change. Later we discovered that the low caloric intake actually countered the positive effects of the exercise program, and we began to encourage normal eating patterns, controlling only the type of food that was eaten. It was increasingly apparent that dieting was ineffective and dangerous and thus actually made obesity worse.

Encouraged by the success we were experiencing, we developed almost a missionary zeal to get the ideas out to the public. We began a series of weight-control seminars in which we lectured on the various aspects of the system. It soon became clear that the information was too complex to be presented in a short half-day seminar, so we began writing our ideas down so that they would be available for reference after the seminar as well as to those who could not attend the seminars. In our zeal to include all we had learned, we soon had reams of paper filled with very complex ideas. Realizing that this material could never be used in its voluminous state, we began to carefully pare it down to the "nitty gritty" that now makes up chapters one through five. The most important parts of the leftover material were placed in the appendices for those of you who wish to expand your understanding. We also included a rather large list of references relating to these new ideas for the serious student who reads our book.

Although there was little support for these ideas in the lay literature when we first started, many magazines have written articles regarding "setpoint" theory. In fact, a beautifully written book entitled *Dieters Dilemma* by Bennett and Gurin came on the market just as we were finishing our first draft of the book. These authors had obviously read the same scientific literature that we had and had come to the same conclusions. Their work provides to the skeptical a great deal of proof for our ideas. However, these writers are not clinicians and they make no suggestions for treatment except that exercise seems to be helpful.

Other writers have picked up some of the ideas and have written about the effectiveness of exercise or the futility of dieting. However, they usually don't put it all together. Any diet that doesn't provide all the body's needs will merely interfere with the desired long-term changes.

One of the advantages of our plan is that the same food and eating suggestions are made for all phases of weight management. Since your weight will automatically stabilize at some new constant level, there is no need for a special stabilization plan, and a different set of maintenance principles. We are also delighted that the dietary suggestions we use for this new program are the same as we would give for overall optimal health. The foods we recommend can and should be eaten by the entire family and should, in fact, greatly improve their nutritional status. We also emphasize exercise and know that it is critical not only for weight control, but also for health.

We can think of very few medical conditions that would be harmed by these suggestions. Those taking medication for high blood pressure or diabetes (either insulin or pills) should be followed closely by their physician as both of these conditions usually improve very quickly, and it becomes necessary to reduce or even completely stop the medication. However, anyone on a special diet for health reasons should check with his doctor before starting this system. Anyone who is over 35 years old, who is grossly obese, or who has musculoskeletal or other serious health problems should consult with a doctor before starting the outlined exercise program.

In the near future, we believe that knowledgeable people will no longer use reduced caloric diets for weight management. We also believe that others will write books and articles based on these principles as the principles become more widely known. Although the approach may differ, they are here to stay.

We are appalled by the widespread ignorance about effective weight management; by the extreme, dangerous methods that are being used, and by the number of people who have damaged their health and produced problems and sorrow for themselves through unwise dietary practices. We hope that this book will help many to give up destructive dieting behavior and become healthy again.

Acknowledgement

We express appreciation to Janell Tyson and Trixie Hicken Bellows who typed — and retyped — the manuscript. And to Dr. Glade Hunsaker whose counsel and direction kept us on track as we reorganized the mass of material into a readable product. We wish to thank Jolayne Remington, Joyce Nixon (J. N.), and Mariteresa Bergeron (M. B.) who have provided most of the recipes. We also thank our wives who saw so little of us during the final phases of preparation. And a special thanks to our patients and friends who willingly tried our new ideas and proved they work.

Notes to the 12th Printing

Since this book was first published seven years ago, a great deal of new information that supports our concepts has become available. One of the most interesting involved research that evaluated the diets of more than 800 women and that was reported in *The New*

England Journal of Medicine.[1] After twelve years, it was found that the women who had died from stroke-associated causes ate an average of 361 calories per day *less* than the other women in the study.

If what we've always heard about calories was true, these women should have lost more than thirty-five pounds a year. Instead, they were actually fatter than the other women in the study! The conclusion? Overweight people consistently eat less than thin people. Researchers believe that if these stroke victims had boosted their intake of potassium by eating just one fresh fruit or vegetable serving a day, their chances of dying would have been cut by 40 percent!

The food recommendations made in this book are sound, healthy ones. The American Heart Association, the American Cancer Society, and a number of other groups have made similar recommendations. Why? We now know that the protective vitamins, minerals, and other chemical substances found in food can help prevent cancer and heart disease—if they are eaten in adequate amounts. Restricting the amount of food you eat will not only make you fatter, but it will cause or contribute to cancer, hypertension, heart disease, diabetes, and other diseases we once thought were caused by obesity. The traditional treatment—cutting calories—is more dangerous than being overweight!

The plan for weight management in this book will enable you to eat plenty of protective nutrients—probably more than you have eaten in years—while still losing weight. If you find that reading the book isn't enough, there are other helps available. *Recipes to Lower Your Fat Thermostat* features more than 400 recipes that are suitable for the plan outlined here. A new audiotape series, *The New Neuropsychology of Weight Control,* explains the program in a way that will help you follow the basic concepts—and the companion videotape, *The Will to Change,* will further inspire and motivate you. The colored pages at the end of this book give complete ordering information.

Ready to get on the road to a more healthy lifestyle that will help you achieve your weight goals? Start reading!

1.Kay-Tee Khaw and Elizabeth Barrett-Connor, Dietary Potassium and Stroke-Associated Mortality, *The New England Journal of Medicine,* Jan. 29, 1987, Vol. 316, No. 5, pp. 235-240.

Chapter One
Why Diets Don't Work

Dieting is not effective in controlling weight; it has never worked, and it never will. Admittedly, you can get temporary weight loss with a diet, but each scheme ultimately gives way to weight gain, and subsequent losses become increasingly difficult. You become hungrier and more obsessed with food, frequently eating out of control. You get tired and weak, have poor endurance, and generally feel awful about yourself; worst of all you get progressively fatter on less and less food.

Dieting actually makes you fatter! Some 200-pound women have said, "If I didn't diet all the time, I would be 300 pounds." The truth is, if they had never dieted, they would probably weigh less than 150 pounds, and if they don't stop dieting, they may soon weigh their feared 300 pounds.

The whole concept of dieting to lose weight is based on wrongheaded concepts. For many years, the scientific community has blamed overeating for all fatness and has suggested dieting as the cure: All you have to do is eat less food than your body needs and automatically the body will use the excess fat; weight loss will naturally follow. Although the idea seems theoretically correct, it simply doesn't work. The truth is that excess body fat has relatively little to do with the amount of food eaten. Instead, it seems clear that body fat is actually regulated by a control center in the brain referred to as the weight-regulating mechanism, which actually "chooses" the amount of body fat that it considers ideal for our needs and then works tirelessly to defend that level.

This fat level (and thus the weight level) that the weight-regulating mechanism "chooses" is called the "setpoint" and can be compared to the thermostat in a home. If the thermostat is set at 70 degrees (setpoint), the furnace will be activated when the temperature falls below the setpoint temperature to maintain the desired heat level. In a similar way, the weight-regulating mechanism directs the body to maintain the setpoint weight when dieting threatens its stability (see appendix 1 and 10 for further details).

This weight-regulating mechanism controls body weight in two critically important ways. First, it has a profound influence on the amount of food that you eat, dramatically increasing or decreasing your appetite as needed to maintain the setpoint weight. Second, it can actually trigger systems in the body to "waste" excess energy if you overeat, or to "conserve" energy if you eat too little.

This dominating mechanism that controls eating can be compared to the breathing controls. You have no control over the "need" to breathe, but you can override breathing to speak, swim, or blow into a musical instrument. However, if you hold your breath for too long, the drive to breathe will become so strong that you can no longer continue to control it.

The weight-regulating mechanism functions in a similar manner. Based on the nutritional needs of the body, you get a message to eat. While you have absolutely no control over the eating drive, you do have control over how you handle that drive. You decide when to eat, what to eat, and how much to eat. If you consistently eat less than your setpoint demands, the drive to eat may become so strong that the conscious, decision-making part of you will no longer be in control, causing you to eat quantities and kinds of food that will nudge the setpoint higher (see appendix 2).

The weight-regulating mechanism can also direct systems in your body to either conserve or waste energy. These systems have been poorly understood in the past, but now it is easy to see why some people can eat very little and still remain fat while others eat a lot but don't gain an ounce. As scientists, we have never been able to explain this paradox until we became aware of how these systems work.

The first system, surprisingly, is regulated by the amount of food you eat; large intakes increase the rate at which you burn calories while restricted intakes decrease this rate. The second system involves a different kind of fat called "brown fat." Brown fat is different from the "storage" fat in that it has the ability to burn part of the food you eat and waste the excess energy as heat so it doesn't have to be stored as fat. People who can eat large quantities of food without gaining weight use brown-fat activity to waste some of this extra energy. People who have weight problems have little brown fat activity.

A third system involves a cellular "pump" that repeatedly pumps sodium and potassium across the cell membranes of billions of cells in the body. This pump uses energy and is driven by an enzyme called sodium-potassium ATP-ase. Thin people have much higher levels of sodium-potassium ATP-ase than the obese and can therefore waste excess energy much more easily (see appendix 3).

Recognizing the important role of these energy-conserving and energy-wasting systems in weight control, we now understand why restricted diets don't work; you decrease the amount you eat in an effort to lose weight, and the body slows down its metabolism to protect its fat stores. The less you eat, the less you burn. And although you may lose some weight initially, you soon level off and wonder why you don't continue to lose. At the same time, the body makes other metabolic, hormonal, and enzymatic changes to conserve energy, leaving you lethargic, tired, and unable to maintain a normal activity level.

This decrease in activity leads to other problems for the dieter. First, decreased activity raises the setpoint, which further stimulates a vicious cycle of increased hunger and energy conservation. Second, it causes a loss of muscle tissue so that less fat can be burned. Third, it even affects your response to insulin which causes an increased fat storage. No wonder many frustrated heavy people retain their weight despite diets of 1,000 calories per day! We now understand that attempting to correct weight problems with reducing diets is like bailing out leaking boats. Water keeps pouring in no matter how effectively you bail. Repeated bailing can even make the holes bigger and the problems worse. To be stopped, the leaks must be found and repaired. Successful treatment of a weight problem requires the same approach: find the basic problem and treat it.

In the same sense, it is also easy to see why some people never gain weight. If energy-wasting mechanisms are working effectively, excess calories are "wasted" and fat stores remain constant.

The critical question, then, is why the setpoint is so high in some and so low in others. Throughout past generations, the amount of body fat has often been critical for survival. Physically fit and very mobile ancestors enjoyed low setpoints because they were forced to travel great distances to capture food and to escape danger. On the other hand, a high setpoint with its large fat stores and its ability to conserve energy conferred survivability to ancestors whose environment dictated severe seasonal food shortages and famines fatal to their thinner contemporaries.

Although it is likely there are at least some genetic tendencies to have either a high setpoint with its overfat body or a low setpoint with its lean body, fortunately you are not permanently "stuck" with an undesirable setpoint level. Just as your ancestors developed the ability to store or waste energy depending on the survival needs of the environment, you too can change or "reprogram" your setpoint by the lifestyle choices you make each day (see appendix 4 for a more detailed discussion of factors contributing to obesity).

For instance, exercise is a most critical factor in weight control. Inactivity is always detrimental. With a high activity level, the weight-regulating mechanism seems to sense the need for high mobility, the setpoint is lowered, and fat stores are "willingly" given up to produce a more streamlined, easier-to-move body.

Another major factor that affects the setpoint is the type of food eaten. High-fat foods and refined carbohydrates (especially sugar) increase hunger and, if eaten regularly, actually raise the setpoint. This response is almost as if the body anticipates hard times ahead, senses that these high-energy foods can easily be converted into fat, and consequently signals for increased fat storage for survival. Whatever the reason, the setpoint goes up, and you are distressed as you continue putting on weight.

Even dieting, missing meals, and irregular eating trigger the "starvation defenses." The body starts making changes to conserve energy and protect the fat. Often the level of the setpoint is raised as if to provide greater fat stores that offer better protection for the next time starvation conditions exist.

Understanding these factors has made it possible to develop treatment principles that really work. Patients who have tried for years to lose weight using conventional approaches are amazed at how they can effectively lose weight while eating more food than they have eaten for many years. Hunger comes under control. Patients report thinking less and less about food, being able to eat in better control, losing cravings and the desire to binge. They have much more energy. They feel more like exercising and it is easier for them to keep on a good exercise program. They seem to increase their fitness level more quickly. After the first few weeks of adjustment, they feel calmer and more relaxed and are more emotionally even-keeled. They feel better about themselves and are often less depressed. Many health problems like headaches, high blood pressure, and intestinal problems dramatically improve. Most people report feeling "great" or "wonderful," better than they have felt in years.

Comparing the traditional weight-loss approaches to the findings of our research reminds us of the fable called The Wind and the Sun. The Wind and the Sun had an argument as to who was the stronger. They decided on a contest to settle the issue. The one who could remove the coat from the traveller walking the road below would be the winner. The Wind tried first. The initial blast almost stripped the coat from the traveller, but he managed to hang onto it and wrap it more securely around himself. As the Wind blew more fiercely, the traveller clutched the coat more firmly to his body and the Wind finally gave up. Taking his turn, the Sun increased his heat. The traveller, becoming hotter and hotter, sensed that the coat was excessive for his needs and took it off.

The traditional approach to weight control, like the wind, may at first partly remove the protective fat, but the body quickly senses danger and "hangs" onto the fat tenaciously. With the reprogramming plan, the body is given a sense of security. Deciding that its needs are not well served by excess fat, it sheds it.

Approaching the Problem

We will present some exciting new treatment principles in the following chapters. Using them will allow your body to "willingly" shed its excess fat.

Beginning with chapter 2 we will discuss the "secrets" of effective exercise for weight control, learning how to use activities to make maximum setpoint changes. Chapter 3 details the problems of a high-fat/high-sugar diet and tells how to change the diet to readjust the setpoint. Since most obese people are irregular eaters who have dieted for much of their lives, one of the major recommendations in Chapter 3 is to eat regularly (and at least sometimes to satiety) to avoid the starvation defenses discussed above. An evaluation system will be presented in Chapter 4, helping you evaluate your progress and understand the principles more thoroughly. The final chapter will help you set realistic goals. Because there are so many variations of body build, many of you never will completely fit the "idealized" mold you see in fashion magazines. In this chapter you will measure your level of body fat and compute your ideal body weight based on specific calculations.

Appendices are also included to present additional information about the basic treatment principles. Included are other factors that affect the setpoint, evidence for the weight-regulating mechanism, a model of the WRM, basic principles of nutrition, meal preparation guidelines and recipes, and basic nutritional values of foods.

We are excited about this system because it lowers the setpoint and changes many of the metabolic, enzymatic, and hormonal problems that keep people fat. Bodies effectively programmed to store and protect excess fat may now be programmed to maintain a naturally lower weight level, and the new body weight will stay down easily and naturally.

For too long people have been trying to "blow" excess fat off their unwilling bodies. The time has come to use a more effective method—one that will by gentle persuasion convince the body to shed its excess fat naturally. We wish you success as you use these principles to lower your setpoint and lose weight naturally.

Chapter Two
The Magic of Exercise

Exercise is the most critical of the factors involved in the weight-control process. The other major factor, eating the proper type of food, will never be effective by itself. You will continue to be unsuccessful in controlling weight until you exercise properly and on a regular basis.

Why Exercise?

If exercise is absolutely essential, why don't more people do it? Regrettably, there are several rather prominent obstacles.

- Finding time: Selecting and retaining a regular exercise time is very difficult; some other demand on your time always seems to have a higher priority.
- Hard work: Although good for you and important, exercise requires energy and makes you tired. Most of you would rather find some method that seems easier and takes less physical effort. Moreover, exercising sometimes seems more like work than fun.
- Slower weight loss: With exercise, muscles sometimes increase in size (especially if you have been inactive). This increase in muscle mass may counter the decrease in fat, and body weight may actually change very little during the initial stages.

Furthermore, the value of exercise has, unfortunately, been underrated and misunderstood. For instance, most people mistakenly think that exercise increases appetite to the point that extra food intake negates the number of calories used. This factor has been clearly proven incorrect. Many people are also discouraged because of the small number of calories used in relation to the effort put out. If the only value of exercise were using calories, the argument would have some credibility; for indeed, it takes a lot of effort to use enough calories to lose even a pound of fat. For instance, walking uses about five calories a minute. Since there are 3500 calories in a pound of fat, you would have to walk about 11½ hours to lose a pound. However, there are a number of compelling reasons to exercise. Of chief importance is that fact that exercise is essential in lowering the setpoint. It also increases the metabolic rate, maintains the muscle mass, increases the enzymes that burn fat, changes the body's chemistry, and makes you feel good. Each of these factors will be discussed in order to emphasize the importance of beginning an exercise program at once and sustaining it for the rest of your life.

Lowering the setpoint. The first and most important reason to exercise is to readjust the setpoint of the weight-regulating mechanism. The fact that exercise performs this role can be seen clearly in the animal world where wild animals are both active and lean. When placed in cages, however, they inevitably get fatter. Similar changes are seen in people who are assigned desk jobs after having been physically active eight hours a day. The body seems to sense that a mobile person (or animal) needs to be thin.

A decrease in fat always occurs as a result of regular exercise, but the amount of loss varies from person to person. For instance, we have found a marked difference in overall percent fat changes among various people who make essentially the same changes in exercise and diet. If you have a higher than normal fat cell number, you may have to exercise much longer and control the type of food you eat much more carefully to get the same reduction in total fat. Although there is no doubt that the percent fat will decrease, the extent of the decrease depends on the person.

There is also a difference in the time it takes to move the setpoint. Some patients begin to change almost immediately. Others may take several months. This factor seems related to the length of time the weight problem has existed and the amount of exercise done weekly.

One lady, a former state beauty queen, exercised for nearly a year in an adult fitness program before major changes in body composition occurred. However, she was exercising only 20 minutes a day, three times a week. A college-aged girl experienced the same problem while exercising three days a week. When she increased to a daily program of about an hour a day, the "mechanism" seemed to come "unstuck" and she experienced satisfactory weight loss. This may seem somewhat discouraging, but these two ladies had long-time weight problems and realized success for the first time in their lives by exercising faithfully. Those who exercise properly and regularly do decrease their fat.

Increasing Resting Metabolic Rate. Another important role of exercise is that it causes the metabolic furnace to burn at a higher level. It is difficult for the body to conserve energy if you are exercising regularly. Even moderate exercise increases the metabolic rate three to eight times. There is even a residual effect from a bout of exercise that keeps the metabolic rate high for several hours following exercise. All of these factors play a role in the basic metabolic activity of the body and make the exerciser a high-calorie consumer whose body is ready and able to waste excess energy at any time. This is a far cry from the energy conservative obese person who sits quietly and walks slowly—conserving energy in every action.

Maintaining Lean Body Mass. Dieting without exercise has one serious drawback: you may lose as much lean muscle tissue as you do fat. Here is what happens. Low caloric intakes often trigger a body process called gluconeogenesis (the process of converting protein to glucose). This process actually breaks down muscle tissue to be used for energy in the place of sugar. Because of this, a person who loses 20 pounds of weight from dieting will often lose as much as 10 pounds of muscle. Of course, this looks good on the scales because total weight is coming off, but any muscle loss decreases the ability to burn fat.

In the body, both carbohydrates and proteins can be changed to fat and stored. However, fat cannot be changed to any other product. The only way fat can be removed from fat cells is to be burned in the muscles for energy. If muscle mass is decreased through dieting, some of the capacity to burn fat is lost.

Exercise may actually increase muscle mass. Most people have seen the effect of a cast on the muscles of an arm or a leg—they appear to have shrunk and become smaller because of the inactivity of the limb while it was in the cast. Likewise, many of you have lost muscle mass from your body because of inactivity. When you begin to exercise, you may get an increase in that lost tissue and become better fat burners. That's the good news. The bad news is that the increased muscle tissue may actually weigh more than the fat that was lost. This is a fairly common initial occurrence associated with exercise, and, if understood, should not cause discouragement. Within a few weeks this stable muscle mass will actually accelerate fat loss. Contrary to the typical diet plan with its rapid initial weight loss (due to loss of muscle tissue and water), with exercise the fastest weight loss may occur later on, when the muscle mass stops increasing and the fitness level is up. Under these conditions you burn more calories with exercise because of the increased muscle mass and because of the increased fitness level, and you enjoy all the other changes associated with exercise as well.

Increasing Fat-Burning Enzymes.

Both fats and carbohydrates are "burned" in the muscles for energy. Each has a separate metabolic pathway that depends on very specific enzymes for the burning to take place. Using a technique called a "muscle biopsy," scientists can take a small piece of muscle tissue and analyze it to see the effect of exercise on the enzymes in these pathways. When biopsies from endurance athletes are compared to those of untrained college students, it can be seen that the athletes have a greater number of fat-burning enzymes. Study has also shown that untrained people could increase those same enzymes by doing any endurance-type exercise for several months. Apparently, in well-trained people, the body "beefs up" the metabolic systems to burn fat more efficiently, protecting the sugar (glucose) in the blood and muscle tissue.

This change can be very important for a person who is trying to control amounts of fat. Remember that you cannot get rid of fat except by burning it in the muscles. Not only will exercise give more muscle, but it will also provide more enzymes to burn the fat. Picture a molecule of fat being released from a fat cell at the beginning of an exercise period (see figure 2.1). If there is sufficient muscle tissue that needs energy, and the muscle cell has fat-burning enzymes, the fat particle will move into the muscle and be burned. On the other hand, if a person has a decreased muscle mass because of dieting, and few enzymes for fat metabolism because of inactivity, the fat particle will simply float around the system for a while, then return to a fat cell for storage.

Figure 2.1

Journey of Fat

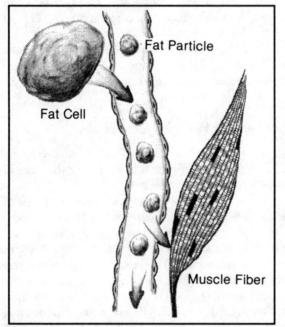

Changing the Body's Chemistry. Insulin is a hormone that is essential for getting sugar into the cell so it can be burned for energy. However, excess insulin can actually cause increased fat storage. Most obese people have excessive insulin because their cells seem to be resistant to it and the body produces more to overcome this resistance. One of the positive effects of exercise is that it increases the responsiveness of cells to insulin. (See appendix 2 for a complete discussion of the role of insulin in fat storage.)

Other hormones are affected, too. Stress-related hormones (like adrenalin and cortisol) are actually metabolized by exercise. This decreases their effect on fat storage. Endorphines, small morphine-like chemicals, are also secreted in the brain as a result of endurance exercise. Endorphines can cause a feeling of well-being and alleviate depression. This decreases the stress levels in most people and may affect fat storage.

The Overall Feeling of Well-being. One of the most important aspects of an exercise program is the way it makes you feel. The more you do, the more you will want to do, and this positive cycle will continue as you lose weight and become more fit. This total increase in activity will accelerate all the other beneficial effects discussed above, and the weight-control process will be enhanced. Mental outlook on life will also improve and feelings of depression will leave. Surely, exercise is a must for anyone who is serious about successful long-term weight control.

How to Exercise for Weight Control

Many people do sit-ups, push-ups, and other muscle-toning exercises each day to decrease fat. Others use rollers or other machines to massage or vibrate fatty areas. Some even wear wide plastic belts or plastic suits to increase heat in the fat areas of the body. All of these approaches are vain. Sit-ups and push-ups are fine for toning the muscles under the fat, but research has shown clearly that "spot reducing" simply does not work. Fat cannot be "bounced" out of a fat cell, nor can it be sweated out. The body stimulates the release of fat from fat cells with little regard for which muscles are doing the work. The best exercises, then, are those that involve the most muscle tissue. The following rules or guidelines for exercise are known to be effective for decreasing the amount of fat in the fat cells and increasing the cardiovascular or endurance fitness of the body.

1. Type of activity. To be successful in burning fat you should use large-muscle rhythmic activity for a long period of time. Some examples of this type of activity are walking, jogging, swimming, jumping rope, bicycle riding, aerobic dancing, bouncing on a minitramp, and hiking. A more complete discussion of various activities with their advantages and disadvantages can be found in appendix 5.

Any of these activities may be used because they involve the large muscles of the hips and legs and can be done continuously for long periods of time. This factor is critical to the success of the program because the metabolic and enzymatic changes discussed will not occur unless you exercise for long, uninterrupted periods of time.

The principle involved here is much like wearing shoes that fit poorly. If you wear them all day, every day for a month, the body will develop a callus to protect the foot. Sporadic wear will have no effect. The same principle applies to exercise — continuous regular exercise will cause changes to occur; sporadic exercise will not.

Straining activities, such as calisthenics or weightlifting, never work. They will strengthen muscles, but they have no effect on the muscle cells in terms of changing the way they burn fat. They are also inferior in terms of total metabolic cost. Rhythmic long-lasting exercise allows much more total work to be done because muscles take turns resting and working, and soon adapt to the stress placed upon them by increasing their ability to use fat.

Sports activities such as tennis, golf, and racquetball are fun, but ineffective in making the enzymatic changes necessary for fat control. Somehow, if you stop and start during your workout, or if you work at very high intensities for short periods and then chase a ball or rest, the body does not feel a need to change metabolically.

2. Intensity. Activity for weight control must be done at a moderate intensity to produce the best results. Many people believe that if it doesn't hurt, they are not benefitting from the activity. This idea is completely false. As mentioned before, the body has separate pathways for metabolizing fat and sugar. Which pathway you use depends upon how hard you work. High-intensity activity uses the sugar pathway almost exclusively, but moderate-intensity activity stimulates the use of fats and the muscular changes associated with that use. Basketball is a good example of the wrong type of activity in terms of intensity. Basketball players either run at a very high speed or stand for foul shots or time-outs. They develop their anaerobic or sugar pathways. These pathways are used specifically for developing large quantities of energy for short periods of time. Little fat can be burned in this system. Although these athletes become well conditioned for basketball, they don't make the changes needed for effective weight control. Obviously, a person who wants to control fat would be better off developing metabolic systems that burn fat and that stimulate muscle changes that aid the process.

One way to tell if you are working too hard is to pay attention to your breathing rate. If you are breathing too hard to carry on a conversation during exercise, you are probably hyperventilating. This is a sure sign that you should slow down. Heavy breathing always occurs when you start using sugars as the primary source of energy.

Another way to tell if you are working at the correct intensity (moderate) is to check your pulse during exercise. You can check it on the inside of the wrist just up from the thumb, or on either side of your Adam's apple in the neck.

Try checking the pulse for 10 seconds right now. The resting pulse will probably be between 10 and 15 beats per 10 seconds (60 to 90 beats per minute). You should use a 10-second count because that will increase your accuracy during exercise. Figure 2.2 shows how the heart rate responds to exercise.

Figure 2.2
10-Second Pulse Count

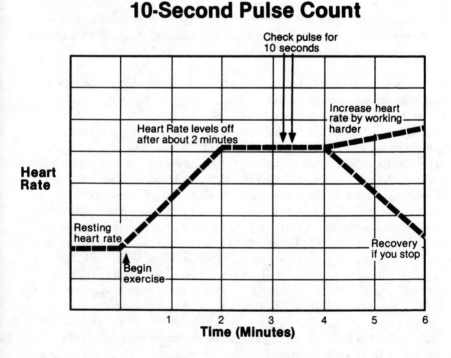

When you begin to exercise, the pulse rate goes up rather quickly and then levels off. To find out your pulse rate during exercise, you should stop and immediately count the pulse for 10 seconds before it comes down too much, then begin walking again. Table 2.1 shows the 10-second heart rate guideline for most people according to age. You should choose a heart rate according to age in the first column (the "70% of maximum" column) when beginning your exercise program. For example, if you are 30 years old, you should exercise at whatever intensity it takes to get a 10-second heart rate of approximately 22 beats. If you count a much higher heart rate, you should decrease the work level; if you count a lower one, increase it. The heart rate actually acts as a speedometer for exercise intensity and helps adjust the exercise efforts to be in harmony with your fitness level.

Table 2.1

10 Second Heart Rate Guideline

Age	(for people who have not exercised much— 70% of maximum)	(for people who have exercised for a while— 80% of maximum)
20	23	27
30	22	25
40	21	24
50	20	23
60	19	21
70	17	20

We have included two heart rate columns because as you get more fit, you can use a higher percentage of maximum heart rate and still receive the benefits of "moderate" exercise.

Remember, these heart rates are guidelines to help you work at a moderate, comfortable pace. If the exercise heart rate is 21 beats for 10 seconds and you are breathless at that intensity, you should slow down. On the other hand, if you can exercise comfortably at a slightly higher heart rate than is listed on table 2.1, work at the higher level.

After checking the intensity by heart rate a few times, you will be aware of how the body feels at the proper intensity and will be able to exercise at that level from then on. The key is to avoid feeling sick when you finish the exercise bout; you should be invigorated and not completely fatigued. You should train, not strain.

Many people fail to establish a regular exercise habit because they overdo when they begin and create an unpleasant exercise experience for themselves. Quite typical of this is the experience of D.R. While in medical school, a best-selling exercise book gave him an enthusiasm for running. The book suggested running a mile and a half as fast as possible to measure fitness. Being somewhat competitive, he overexerted himself and felt terrible. Each workout was also a disaster because he tried to go too fast and too far so that he could be higher on the charts. Needless to say, he was unsuccessful in his attempt to get fit. Later, he started a moderate exercise program using his heart rate as a guide. This program was comfortable and positive, and a regular pattern was established. Overexertion with exercise can cause headaches, nausea, weakness, and shakiness, as well as symptoms of sore muscles, cramps, joint pain, shinsplints, and other musculoskeletal injuries. You should start at a low level and increase carefully if you wish to establish a successful exercise pattern.

Duration of Exercise. Most people exercise too briefly to really get benefits in terms of weight control. The ideal duration is from 45 minutes to an hour a day. Of course, you should begin with a more moderate duration-say 20 minutes. But keep it in the back of your mind to increase to that hour-a-day goal as you become more fit.

Most people can begin at about 20 minutes the first day without any problem. If you choose walking as the exercise mode, you should walk for 10 minutes and then come back. The distance is unimportant.

After walking 20 minutes a day for the first week, you should increase the duration to 25 minutes a day. Again, simply walk for 12 1/2 minutes away from your house and 12 1/2 minutes back. If all goes well the second week at 25 minutes a day, you should increase to 30 minutes a day for the third week. You can increase the duration by five minutes each week until you are up to 60 minutes a day.

If you are young and not too overweight, you may be able to increase the duration more rapidly (e.g., increasing by 10 minutes each week). If older and/or extremely overweight, you may be better off to increase the duration more slowly (e.g., five minutes a day every two or three weeks).

You should not be in too big a hurry to increase duration. If you have been inactive for some time and have extra weight, it will take a while for the musculoskeletal system to toughen up. However, if you are already walking and have been walking for two or three months, you may wish to introduce short periods of jogging during your walk. The pulse should be checked if there is a question about intensity.

If you are using an exercise bike, you may not be able to get the heart rate up for several weeks because of weak leg muscles. You shouldn't worry about this. You should be certain to maintain the proper duration according to the guidelines, and the intensity will come later. It is more important to get the total duration at first than to be at the proper intensity. Activities such as jumping rope may cause the heart rate to go up too high, too rapidly. If this occurs, you should jump for only a short time (until you begin to breathe hard) and then walk around until you feel recovered. You should keep this up until you have completed the proper duration.

Remember, whatever exercise you choose, it must be continuous for the entire duration to make the changes you want to make.

Frequency of Exercise. The last basic rule is to exercise regularly. Developing measureable changes in the cardiovascular system requires that you exercise at least three times a week or every other day. Making changes in a "sticky" setpoint may demand daily exercise. One young lady exercised three times a week for three months and made no change in her weight. After two weeks of daily exercise (for an hour a day) her weight began to decrease, and she reached her ideal weight within three months. Others have shown the same tendency. Exercising daily seems to be much more effective than exercising every other day for problem-weight loss.

Once the ideal weight is reached, exercise frequency can often be decreased with no ill effect. One lady exercised daily until she reached her ideal weight and then got busy and missed exercising for several weeks without experiencing weight gain. Another lady was forced to exercise daily almost four years after losing her problem weight. If she stopped exercising, her weight began to climb. You should exercise daily until you reach your goal; then you can experiment with frequency and duration.

The Aerobic Training Effect

Perhaps the best examples of how exercise affects the setpoint are seen in the long-distance runner, the cross-country skier, or the long-distance bicycle rider. These athletes seem to make all of the changes that can occur in the body to promote very minimum fat levels. Most get their body fat percentage down to about 3 to 5 percent. They all use ideal types of exercise at the right intensity for the proper length of time to make these changes. If they train for an hour a day, they may maintain a fat content of 7 or 8 percent while eating anything they please. If they increase the duration to 1 1/2 or 2 hours per day, still eating as much as desired, the fat level will fall to something like 3 to 5 percent. After competition, when they slack off to a mere one hour per day, the fat content will then return to its previous 7 or 8 percent level.

We are not sure what factors are involved in keeping the setpoint at such a low level in the endurance athlete. It could be the total length of time spent exercising, the total number of calories consumed, the level of fitness achieved, the level of fat-burning enzymes that are developed, or a combination of these factors, or possibly other factors which are yet unknown. But whatever it is that changes the setpoint for these athletes can change yours also.

An example of this effect was seen when a teenage girl who had unsuccessfully tried many weight-reduction programs lost weight spontaneously to a very attractive level. When asked why she was successful this time she replied that she had no idea, since she had made no effort to diet. Closer questioning revealed that she had obtained a dog about six months previously and had been faithfully taking the dog out for long walks each day. This activity was regular enough, long enough, and intense enough to produce the necessary aerobic training effect. This changed the setpoint to a lower level, allowing for natural weight loss.

It would be nice to know exactly how to change the setpoint to a lower level with an absolute minimum of effort. However, since that information is not known at the present time, we must utilize what is known to be effective in producing the aerobic training effect.

Chapter Three
Eat and Get Thin

The traditional role of food in the weight-control process has been limited almost entirely to its caloric content. You have all been taught that eating "too much" brings fat and that losing weight requires decreasing caloric intake. However, an understanding of the weight-regulating mechanism and how it functions dramatically alters the role of food.

In the preceding chapters, you have learned that the body can either waste excess energy if you eat "too much," or conserve energy if you eat too little, to maintain the setpoint weight. Because of this, in the weight-control process, caloric number is simply not as important as are the types of food eaten.

A group of scientists almost accidentally discovered that obesity could be induced in rats by feeding them modest quantities of what is now referred to as the "supermarket diet." This diet is composed of high-fat, high-sugar goodies such as peanut butter, cookies, salami, marshmallows, and similar foods.

Although it is tempting to think that the rats got fat because the food tasted so good that they simply ate too much, some extremely creative experiments have shown that these rats got fat because of the types of food they ate and not because of the amount. Apparently, continually eating fats and sweets raises the setpoint. Once the setpoint is raised, the body stimulates hunger and conserves energy until the new setpoint weight is reached.

A recent study substantiates this idea. Dr. Larry Oscai and his colleagues at the University of Illinois (Chicago), fed two groups of rats exactly the same number of calories for a 60 week experimental period. One group ate regular rat chow (a low fat, high fiber food), and the other ate a diet similar to the typical American diet; that is, about 40% of the calories coming from fats and 25% from sugar. Despite a similar caloric intake, carcass fat averaged 51% for the rats eating the fat–rich diet but only 30% for the rats eating regular rat chow. This study clearly demonstrates that sever obesity can develop in the absence of overeating by simply eating too much fat.

In this chapter, we will present food-intake guidelines that will help you reprogram the setpoint to a lower level. The first three are:

- decreasing fat consumption,
- decreasing refined carbohydrates,
- increasing complex carbohydrates.

These three guidelines are meal related, and following them will lower your setpoint and improve the quality of your diet. The other two guidelines relate to drinking habits. Most overweight people drink too many high-calorie or sweetened drinks and too little water. These guidelines will help you change this behavior.

We will also discuss the problem of being out of harmony with the eating drives from the weight-regulating mechanism and introduce an eating plan to help increase the sensitivity to these drives. When the setpoint comes down, the body must sense the new signals from the weight-regulating mechanism for effective weight loss to occur.

Food-intake Guidelines

The first three guidelines will help reprogram the setpoint to a new, lower level and will make your diet more healthful. It will take some effort to change the type of food normally eaten, but the effort will be worthwhile.

Guideline no.1 - Decrease Fat Consumption. The average American consumes about 40 percent of his calories in the form of fat. Most nutritionists agree that this level of fat is too high and should be reduced because of the health risks involved. However, the amount of decrease is highly controversial. The recommended level of fat intake varies from the Pritikin diet, which specifies from 5 to 10 percent fat, to the American Heart Association levels of 30 percent. An extremely low–fat diet is difficult to manage and may be rather unpalatable. Because we believe that all dietary suggestions must be practical and livable as well as healthful, we suggest that you reduce your fat intake toward the 20 percent mark. This will cut the fat content of your diet in half but leave the food satisfying and palatable. Besides lowering the setpoint so that your weight can normalize more easily, this change will also decrease the caloric density of the food you eat. This means that the same volume of food will contain significantly fewer calories.

To be successful in lowering the fat intake, you must learn to read "nutrition information labels" on cans and packages to evaluate the fat content of food purchased. The typical label lists the serving size, the number of servings per container, a breakdown of total calories per serving; the number of grams of protein, carbohydrates, and fat; and the milligrams of sodium. Figure 3.1 shows the nutrition information label from a box of Golden Grahams cereal:

Figure 3.1

Serving size ....1 ounce (3/4 cup)
Servings per container 18
1 oz. Golden Grahams
Calories 110
Protein (grams) 2
Carbohydrates (grams) 24
Fat (grams) 1
Sodium, mg 345

The question is: "How much fat does this cereal contain?" To compute the number of calories of fat, you must know that each gram of fat contains nine calories. With Golden Grahams, there is one gram of fat per serving, so each serving contains nine calories from fat. Since there are 110 total calories per serving, about 8 percent of the calories come from fat (9/110 = 8 percent).

Now let's evaluate the percent fat from the nutrition label of a can of Campbell's Cream of Potato soup. (Figure 3.2)

Figure 3.2

Calories 90
Protein (grams) 2
Carbohydrate (grams) 14
Fat (grams) 3

Remember that each gram of fat contains nine calories, so the fat in this soup accounts for 27 calories of the total (3 grams x 9 calories

per gram). The percent fat is 27/90, or 30 percent. You can quite easily decrease your fat consumption by carefully evaluating cans and
boxes before purchasing.

There are many other simple guidelines that can be used to
decrease the amount of fat in the diet. For instance, you can decrease
or omit butter, margarine, spreads, or mayonnaise (all of which are
extremely fatty) from sandwiches and bread. You can also decrease
the amount of salad dressing on salads — most are very fatty. Lemon
juice, vinegar, or diet dressings are successful alternatives (check the
percent fat on the label). You should also learn to eat cooked
vegetables without butter or fatty toppings, and raw vegetables
without dips. Vegetables are delicious when prepared properly; you
will soon learn to appreciate their natural flavor.

You must also change the way you prepare foods. Frying
(especially deep-fat frying) increases the amount of fat dramatically.
Many breaded foods (breaded veal cutlets, breaded shrimp, breaded
chicken) are high in fat because they contain not only the natural fat
of the meat but also fat in the breaded exterior, and excess cooking
oil that soaks into the meat as well. Boiling, baking, broiling, barbecuing, microwave cooking, and frying in a Teflon pan without oils all
help decrease the fat content of the foods being cooked.

Deep frying vegetables greatly increases the fat content. For instance, a baked potato is extremely low in fat. When French fried or
made into potato chips it becomes a high fat source. Other vegetables
such as zucchini are also sometimes breaded and deep-fat fried. This
cooking process changes a highly desirable type of food into
something quite undesirable.

Because meat is often a high-fat food, you must eat less if you are
to successfully reduce fat in the diet. You should decrease the total
intake of meat to about 3 1/2 to 4 ounces a day. This can be done by
eating more meatless meals or by reducing the amount of meat consumed with each meal. In reality, the amount of protein required by
the body is not great and can easily be met with almost any diet.
Even vegetarians do well in terms of protein. We are certainly not
suggesting that people become vegetarians, because it is technically
difficult to be a vegetarian and get an optimal diet. However, you can
probably attain most of the benefits of being a vegetarian by merely
reducing the meat to a lower level. Meat should be used more as a
condiment to add flavoring to other foods than as the main-course

serving. For instance, two small pieces of chicken or half a steak might serve to make a meal for an entire family if served Chinese style with rice or stir-fried vegetables. A handful of meat might make a very substantial meal in soup made with staple foods such as beans, rice, barley, lentils, peas, or potatoes.

You can also decrease total fat by emphasizing lower-fat meats such as chicken, turkey, fish, tuna, and lean cuts of beef such as round, flank, and rump. You should avoid meats such as bacon, sausage, ham, hot dogs, lunchmeats, and fatty cuts of beef. The skin from chicken and turkey is high in fat and should be removed before eating. Any visible fat on lean cuts of meat should also be removed.

Another way to decrease the amount of fat in the diet is to use less fat than is called for in recipes. Surprisingly, reducing the oil by half will leave almost no effect on the taste and texture of most foods (breads, muffins, etc.), but the product will be much lower in fat. Most dairy products are high in fat and should be avoided. Skim milk or 1-percent milk has the same protein and vitamin content as regular milk and will taste just as good when you get used to it. Regular cheeses can be replaced by low-fat cottage cheese or skim-milk cottage cheese made at home. Homemade yogurt is also a low-fat dairy product. Most commercial yogurts are high in both fat and sugar. If you have a question about the fat content of any food, check the Composition of Food table in appendix 13.

Guideline no.2 - Reduce Refined Carbohydrates. Most people have acquired a taste for sugar and white flour. Manufacturers of prepared foods take advantage of this taste by using large quantities of sugar in their products. For instance, most breakfast cereals have sugar as either the first or second major ingredient. Of the dozens of boxed cereals, regrettably few have no sugar added.

White flour is also a problem since it is used so extensively in foods. Even many whole-wheat breads contain large quantities of white flour. Sometimes the white flour is given a fancy term such as enriched white flour or fortified flour, but it is still a refined carbohydrate and is likely to affect insulin response and the setpoint.

There are several ways of decreasing the amount of sugar in the diet. Some nutritionists suggest using honey instead of sugar because honey is almost twice as sweet. Therefore, you can cook with less total sweetener and obtain the same basic level of sweetness. Honey, in addition, has a certain amount of fructose or fruit sugar which tends to be absorbed more slowly and may therefore have less effect on insulin than conventional sugar. However, because any advantage of fructose over regular sugar is only minor, you should limit quantities to very low levels. You can also decrease sugar intake by decreasing desserts in the diet. Most desserts are extremely high in both fats and sugars. You can either go "cold turkey" and cut them out altogether or substitute fruit or a good low-fat grain cereal instead. There are also some low-fat, low-sugar dessert recipes available if desserts are important to you. If none of these approaches work, at a minimum you should certainly decrease the size of dessert portions.

Much of the refined carbohydrates you eat come from the habit of snacking. Part of the snacking pattern may be the result of rapidly falling blood sugar levels related to the release of insulin in the body. When you eat excessive sugars, you stimulate the release of insulin, which in turn decreases blood sugar and creates a strong urge to eat within only a few hours of your first sugar intake. Therefore, decreasing sugar intake often reduces the need to snack. Snacking is acceptable if you are hungry, but you should be sure that the snack is a low-sugar food such as vegetables, fruits, whole wheat cereals or breads.

Can artifical sweeteners be used instead of sugar? Although there are no calories in artificial sweeteners, they are not recommended for two reasons. First, artificial sweeteners seem to enhance the desire for sweets, and you may find it difficult to eat good, basic food without sweetening. Luckily, your tastes do change when you decrease the amount of sweets you eat, and foods such as cereals and grapefruit become very palatable. The second problem is that artificial sweeteners may also raise the setpoint.

Guideline no. 3 - Increase Complex Carbohydrates.
Many health experts suggest that the majority of our diet should come in the form of complex carbohydrates. The suggested amount varies from 45 to 80 percent depending on the expert. Complex carbohydrates are found in whole grains, vegetables, and fruits, i.e., whole-grain cereals, brown rice, potatoes, squash, carrots, tomatoes, and apples. These foods should be eaten as they are grown, without processing them to some other form. They are actually composed of

sugars that are linked together in such a way that the breakdown process takes much longer than with simple or refined sugars. Because of this, these foods are very satisfying: they take longer to be broken down, and they produce an even and smooth absorption into the bloodstream. They do not stimulate the large rise in insulin levels with its attendant rapid fall of blood sugar so typical of refined sugar ingestion. (See Figure 3.3 for a comparison between simple and complex carbohydrates.)

Whole-grain cereal and vegetable products are probably the best sources of complex carbohydrates and have been used by most primitive societies for years. Some of these foods such as wheat, rice, beans, peas, lentils, potatoes, and taro provide not only the energy and basic nutrient needs but much of the protein needs as well. Because of nutritionists' emphasis on the need for protein, these foods have often been condemned because they usually lack some essential amino acid. However, recent research has shown that if you eat a variety of different vegetable proteins, you will usually have no difficulty obtaining enough complete protein. This concept is discussed more fully in appendix 6. Fruit contains sugars that are in a more simple form than the sugars found in vegetables and grains. However, the fruit sugars (fructose) are absorbed more slowly than refined sugars (sucrose), and, because they are bound in the cell structure of the plant, are not released as rapidly into the bloodstream. Fruit also contains vitamins that are not as easily obtained from other sources. For these reasons, we classify fruits as complex carbohydrates. However, you should not make fruits the mainstay of your diet since they contain very little protein and lack many of the vitamins and minerals the body really needs.

Guideline no.4 - Decrease Calorie-Containing Fluids. It is extremely common for people to take in more calories than their bodies can successfully waste by drinking high calorie fluids to satisfy thirst. Some people also interpret thirst as hunger and eat when thirsty.

Drinking calorie-containing fluids contributes to obesity in several ways. The sugars (or sweeteners) are absorbed quickly and cause a rapid rise in insulin with all of its negative effects (see Appendix 2). Caffeine drinks (even those without calories) also stimulate insulin production. Liquids require no chewing, are therefore quickly consumed and leave the stomach so rapidly that they provide little lasting satiety. This leads to ingesting more calories than the body can waste, causing excess fat production.

It is critical to decrease the intake of sweet liquids such as soda pop, even if sweetened with artificial sweeteners. When thirsty, you should drink water; if this fails to satisfy you, eat an appropriate snack.

Guideline no.5 - Drink Adequate Amounts of Water.
Many obese people have become insensitive to their thirst drives and eat when their real need is for water. To overcome this basic contributor to obesity, you should learn to drink adequate amounts of water. If uncertain whether a drive represents thirst or hunger, drink a glass of water. If not satisfied with water, you are probably experiencing a hunger drive and should eat some food which requires chewing and will not be digested too quickly. It may take a while to get used to drinking water, but if you persist you should soon become more sensitive to the thirst drive and begin to enjoy normal thirst.

Opinions vary as to how much water is ideal. We feel that six glasses daily are a minimum and that most people should drink more. You should not drink more than 20 glasses unless perspiring profusely and losing excessive fluid. Excess water consumption can cause an increase of antidiuretic hormone, which can produce problems. We have never come across this problem, but routinely encounter people having difficulty drinking enough water.

You may wish to drink several glasses of water with each meal. This will help distend the stomach and signal satiety. Some people think that drinking water with meals dilutes the digestive juices and is therefore bad for digestion. Unless you have had part of the stomach removed because of ulcers or cancer, or a hiatus hernia, there is no reason to restrict water in any way.

For some people, drinking cold water produces nausea or stomach pain. If this is a problem, try drinking warmer water. Some people have trouble drinking water because they don't like the taste and get more enjoyment out of pop, milk, or juice. In these cases, you may wish to try bottled water, use a purification system, or find better tasting water from some nearby area. Persistence will usually allow you to get used to almost any water, regardless of how bad it tastes. The flavor can be altered by drinking it at different temperatures, letting it stand for a while, cooling it with ice, or by adding a few drops of lemon or lime juice.

Guideline no. 6 - Eat in Harmony with the Weight-regulating Mechanism

We have discussed all of the techniques that can be used to lower the setpoint successfully and have pointed out how important this is in the process of controlling weight. However, if not in harmony with the eating drives from the weight-regulating mechanism, you may eat more food than the weight-regulating mechanism "asks" for, and still have problems losing weight. In fact, many of us are overweight because we consistently eat more than our body can waste and maintain a body weight higher than the setpoint. If your weight is higher than setpoint, you could lose weight easily by getting in harmony with the eating drives. This may explain the rapid weight loss in some people resulting from behavior modification. Those who fail to lose weight with behavior modification are probably in harmony with their eating drives and their weight is at the weight level set by the weight-regulating mechanism.

Chronic dieters are perhaps the best example of people who are out of touch with their weight-regulating mechanism. Their weight is usually below the setpoint, but they eat much less than they are "told" to eat by their eating drives. They feel that their weight problem is entirely associated with overeating; that the less they can eat, the better they will lose weight. With this attitude, they feel that hunger is a sign that they are being "good," that they are succeeding and working toward their goal. This "dieter's" mentality places them in a no-win situation. If they don't eat, they may feel good psychologically, but they will feel weak and miserable physically. If they do eat, they feel guilty, angry at themselves, and in despair that they will never succeed. When the drives to eat get strong enough, the resolve they once felt breaks down often resulting in "binge" eating of large quantities of food very quickly, and the food choices are often the very foods the dieter wishes to avoid. Completely out of control, the dieter feels extreme remorse and guilt. The self-image falls further, and the dieter feels the need to diet again — as if dieting were a method of punishment that would help atone for those eating "sins." This binging and starvation regimen is very common among dieters, and we feel it is a very serious obstacle to good mental and physical health: an obstacle that likely raises the setpoint (see Appendix 4).

If you are out of touch with your eating drives, it will be important to "listen" to your body and pay attention to the feelings it gives you relating to food. This may be more difficult than it sounds. Many of you have gotten so used to denying or ignoring the hunger drive that you are no longer sensitive to it.

The question is, how do you get back in touch with your eating drives? First, it is important to eat regularly; at least three times a day. Second, one of these meals should be a "full meal" in which enough food is eaten to produce complete satiety. These two guidelines are so important for learning to eat in harmony with eating drives that we will discuss them in detail.

Eating Plan for Increasing Your Sensitivity to Hunger

The eating drives should become a major factor in the eating behavior. You should eat when hungry and should stop when you receive messages of satisfaction. Since hunger occurs naturally every four to six hours, it is critical to eat regularly so that natural hunger and satiety can be felt. The first meal of the day has sometimes been a problem. However, nutritionists have always stressed the importance of a good breakfast, and we agree with that philosophy. A lack of hunger in the morning could be because the natural drive to eat in the morning has been supressed by missing breakfast for several years or because of the hormonal changes that occur at night to allow sleeping without hunger. Nausea or other unpleasant side effects could be related to the high fat content of the typical breakfast which causes distress in some people.

Some people complain that eating breakfast actually increases their hunger drive during the day. This response may be related to eating too many refined carbohydrates in the morning meal. This can cause rapid sugar absorption and an insulin spike that will yield low blood sugar levels and hunger in a few hours.

If not hungry first thing in the morning, you should probably eat a very light, low-fat breakfast anyway. Eating the right kind of breakfast regularly will soon lead to natural hunger in the morning.

Although there is little direct evidence that breakfast is critical to the weight-loss process, studies comparing "meal skippers" and "regular eaters" show that the meal skippers are fatter,with higher cholesterol levels and more problems with the insulin mechanism. We have also noticed that overweight people seem to skip breakfast more than normal-weight people do. Surely, learning to eat a proper breakfast will be an important step in getting in touch with the eating drives.

You must also be careful to avoid the fat and sugar commonly found in the traditional breakfasts. The following suggestions can be used to create an enjoyable low-fat, low-sugar breakfast:

- Eat a bowl of whole grain sugarless prepared cereal (like puffed wheat, shredded wheat, or grape nuts, without sugar added), served with skim, 1 or 2 percent milk. Have a little fresh fruit such as strawberries or bananas on top or serve with a small glass of juice, half a grapefruit or an orange.
- Prepare whole-wheat porridge (see recipe in wheat section) or other cooked cereal. You may wish to add a small amount of honey for sweetener and serve with fruit or juice.
- Try an egg cooked any way you wish (if fried, be careful of excess fat) served with one or two slices of whole wheat toast lightly buttered or with no butter: serve with fruit or juice.
- A different breakfast could include low-fat cottage cheese with fresh pineapple, strawberries or peaches, and one or two slices of whole wheat toast.
- Make two or three whole-wheat pancakes and serve without butter and with only a very small amount of jam or fruit syrup. Include half a grapefruit or an orange for balance.
- Try a few lightly buttered bran muffins served with any kind of fruit.

Lunch can also be a problem because it is so often eaten at a "fast food" restaurant and most fast-food lunches are high in both fat and sugar (see Appendix 13). The ideal lunch would be mostly complex carbohydrates. They yield greater satiety with fewer calories and will also influence the WRM to a lower level.

Soup can be very satisfying. A recent study showed that eating soup at least once a day caused a weight loss even with no other changes. The more often soup was eaten, the more weight was lost.

Some soups seem to be better than others to induce satiety. Broth soups may not have enough nutrients to be very satisfying. Cream-based soups may have extra fats or refined carbohydrates that are not needed. The best soups are water-based soups with good staple nutrients such as peas, beans, rice, barley or potatoes. Although some of these are a little higher in calories than other soups, the increased satiety value is worth the few extra calories.

You should read the labels on prepared soups and avoid those with high levels of fat or added sugar and avoid a large number of crackers. A slice of homemade bread may be better. (See Appendix 13.)

Sandwiches can also provide an excellent lunch. However, you should choose whole-wheat bread whenever possible and use small portions of low-fat meats with generous cuts of lettuce and tomatoes. You should also avoid high-fat spreads and butter. Some raw vegetables and a piece of fruit with the sandwich will help both nutrition and taste.

Salads are also good for lunch. However, there is so much water and so few calories in lettuce salad that the satiety value is poor and you may feel hungry in a short time even with a large helping. Adding staple foods such as peas, beans, corn or lean meat strips to a salad will enhance the satiety value. A slice of whole wheat bread or other nutritious food along with the salad will also enhance satiety. You should be very careful with salad dressings; they are mostly fats and sugars and have a very high caloric density. One tablespoon of some salad dressings has the same caloric value of one and one-half to two pounds of lettuce.

Both breakfast and lunch (or the evening meal if dinner is at noon) should be "light meals." That is, they should contain only enough food to take away the strong hunger drive. The amount of food required to take away this hunger drive depends on several factors:

- Time since last meal. If you have not eaten for many hours, a relatively large meal may be required before you can comfortably stop eating.
- Prior eating patterns. If you have been a restrained eater, you may have a strong desire to eat.
- Type of food in last meal. If you have eaten sugars with your previous meal or as a snack, you may have a strong hunger

drive because of low blood sugar levels brought about by the strong insulin spike.

All of these situations may make it difficult to eat only a small meal. However, the size of the light meal may not be too critical since you will tend to balance out the calories the next time you eat if you "listen" to your hunger drive.

It is probably a good idea to plan to eat a fixed amount of food. When it is gone, eating should stop. Avoid buffet luncheons or other settings involving unlimited amounts of palatable food; you may be tempted to eat more than you should.

We are not suggesting that you go hungry or disobey the urges of the hunger mechanisms. In fact, the light meal should be satisfying despite the feeling that you could certainly eat more. Within a few minutes you should feel content and not bothered with continued hunger drives. If you are consistently hungry after a light meal, you are probably eating too little. You should remember that the techniques are designed to bring you into harmony with your needs; they are not to hide, mask, deny, or put off needs.

Since a light meal may not produce continued satiety until the next meal, a snack may be useful for controlling excessive hunger and help you get in harmony with the drives of the weight-regulating mechanism. However, you should be careful to snack only in response to real hunger and avoid the tendency to snack for entertainment or pleasure. Any type of food except refined carbohydrates can be used for a snack, as long as it is eaten in small quantities (under 100 calories). The following hints will allow you to use snacks properly:

- Be careful with traditional snacks. Most are high in sugar and/or fat.
- Don't drink a snack. Drink water if you're thirsty.
- If vegetables or fruit don't satisfy, try a slice of homemade bread or a small dish of cereal.
- Avoid high caloric snacks such as dried fruit, raisins, nuts, or peanut butter.
- Drink some water with your snacks to increase the satiety value.

The second major guideline for getting back in harmony with the eating drive relates to eating one "full meal" a day to complete satiety. This suggestion is quite different from the conventional approach, but it is necessary if you ever hope to be successful.

This meal should usually be eaten in the evening to help balance daily requirements and to overcome the tendency to eat during the evening hours. Since there is a prolonged satiety period of four to six hours following a full meal, you should eat this meal at least four hours prior to going to bed. This way, you will be able to enjoy this period when you need it most—while awake and during the time of day when it is most difficult to control eating. If you eat shortly before bedtime, the satiety period is wasted during sleep when it is not really needed. Eating just prior to bedtime may also decrease your ability to sleep. If you are slightly hungry at bedtime, despite having eaten a full meal that night, a small snack might be entirely appropriate. The size and type of snack required to assure optimal comfort and sleep can be determined only through trial and error. You need to become sensitive to the driving forces of the body and live in harmony with them to assure maximal comfort.

If you have eaten properly during the day, the nutrient requirements for the evening meal are only moderate and can be met by a volume of food which can be comfortably contained in the stomach without overdistention. However, if you go all day without eating, you may eat considerably more than the stomach can comfortably hold and feel distressed for a number of hours until the stomach empties to a more comfortable level. Eating only once a day may also make it difficult to satisfy the body's need for nutrients and stimulate a strong desire to eat even when your stomach is full.

For some people, evening may not be the best time to eat the full meal. People working in the evenings and home during the day may find morning or afternoon a better time to eat. Regardless of the situation, you must find a time when the four-to-six hour satiety period works best to help you control the eating drives.

You should continue eating the full meal until you are completely satisfied. You should not stop when the worst of the hunger has subsided. If you stop eating before you are satisfied, the drive from the feeding center will remain; it will become rather insistent later in the evening, and you will probably end up eating more anyway.

Two or more glasses of water should be consumed with the full meal. This will serve to provide part of the body's water needs, plus, help to create the distention of the stomach necessary for satiety with fewer calories.

The full meal should also consist of a reasonable balance of complex carbohydrates, proteins and fats; with the carbohydrate making up about 65 to 80 percent of the total, protein about 10 to 15 percent, and about 10 to 20 percent fat.

The eating and drinking guidelines we have discussed in this chapter are critical because they help lower the setpoint of the weight-regulating mechanism. A lowered setpoint will decrease the eating drive so the body can shed the excess fat.

The eating plan will help you increase your sensitivity to eating drives and allow you to eat just what your body needs to function effectively and at the proper weight. Proper eating also helps you avoid the "starvation defenses" associated with the restricted intake of food. Surprisingly, patients who get in harmony with their eating drives begin to feel more like exercising. It is almost as if the body says it's okay to use energy now that you're eating enough for your needs.

You may have a difficult time accepting these guidelines because you have dieted for so many years and this approach just doesn't feel the same. An article in the December 1982 issue of Woman's Day magazine entitled, "I Quit Dieting and Lost Weight" gave a rare insight to the principles in this chapter. The author quit dieting because none of the "999" diets she had used had helped her lose weight. After a short time, she began to feel like exercising, her weight began to decrease and her clothes felt looser. To her surprise, she lost 50 pounds during the first year and continues to lose weight.

Although she didn't understand the reason for her success, we do. She had inadvertently stumbled on to many of the principles we have outlined in this book. You too can be successful by applying these correct principles.

Figure 3.3

CARBOHYDRATES

SUGAR	VERSUS	**COMPLEX**
Concentrated		Diluted with lots of water and fiber
High calorie density		Low calorie density
Rapid breakdown and absorption — takes only a few minutes		Slow breakdown and absorption — takes hours to digest
Small particles		Large particles — broken down by mechanical action and digestive enzymes — fiber needs to be separated — cell walls must be broken down
Simple molecule — two sugars		Complex molecules — long chains, several thousand sugar molecules long
Split by salivary enzymes		Sugars split from ends of chain in intestines by enzymes from pancreas
Causes rapid rise in blood sugar to high levels		Gradual increase in blood sugar to appropriate levels
Requires large quantities of insulin		Requires small amounts of insulin
No vitamins or minerals		Lots of vitamins and minerals

Chapter Four
Tracking Your Progress

Now that you are aware of the principles of proper weight control, we hope you are excited about starting. You are facing a very sensible weight-reduction system; there are no forbidden foods, no exacting menus to follow, no calories to count, no need to weigh food or measure portions, and no reason to count carbohydrates, fat or protein grams. You will neither have to fight hunger nor resist snacking, and you can eat until you are satisfied. However, the virtues that make this system so practical and livable in the long term may create a short-term dilemma. Most diets are easy to follow for a short time because they tell you exactly what and how much to eat. We could do the same by providing an exact and carefully controlled menu, but this would defeat the entire idea. We feel that it is best for you to select your own foods, learning to eliminate those that cause problems and to eat amounts that are naturally required to satisfy you. If you are somewhat overwhelmed by the foregoing discussion, relax; the following few suggestions will get you on your way.

1) Exercise

Start exercising faithfully; increase duration and intensity gradually. The sooner you start, the more quickly changes will occur. Start today (or at the latest, tomorrow)—in most cases with walking—and the finer details will become clear later.

2) Diet

Do everything suggested. Jump into the whole program; don't dabble your toes around the edge. Do the best you can, but don't try to switch to entirely new types of food. You are more likely to be successful in the long run if you continue to use your same basic foods, altering them to conform to the principles.

3) Don't Expect Perfection

Don't allow yourself to get discouraged or to feel like a failure. Making significant lifestyle changes is not easy, and there is always a tendency to revert to old habit patterns. If you slip, take a deep breath and try again.

4) Be Patient

Excess fat doesn't accumulate overnight, and it won't disappear that quickly either. Although changes may start occurring right away, it may take several months before you notice major changes, and it may take many months until these changes are complete.

If you are a seasoned dieter, you are probably used to seeing quick results in short periods of time. You need to change this attitude. Keep reminding yourself that this is a long-term program; you must be patient.

5) Set Realistic Goals

Many people find goal-setting an effective way to make changes. However, you should not set weight-loss goals since you can't directly control your weight. Set performance goals instead, such as exercising each day or avoiding pop and candy, or attaining 90 or more points from the scoring system presented next in this chapter. These goals are attainable!

A realistic weight goal is also important (see chapter 5). You may be surprised at how close you are to an ideal body weight even though you may be quite distant from the "idealized" weight you chose long ago.

6) Evaluate Your Progress

Most of you need some indication that you are achieving good results before you will persist with a new behavior. The scoring system that follows will likely be very helpful in providing this accountability check.

The Scoring System

We recognize that many of you can easily change your exercise and eating habits using only the information in chapters 2 and 3.

However, we have found that most of our patients accelerate this progress by using a special "scoring" system we have developed for this purpose. This system allows an evaluation of progress in the three major areas introduced in chapters 2 and 3.

- Exercise
- Food and Drink Choices
- Eating Behavior

Let's look at figure 4.1 and analyze this important chart together. Notice that the progress summary chart has on it the major areas mentioned above, their subheadings and the number of points for each. The "scoring tables" for each area are found at the bottom of the chart. Note that 50 points are awarded for exercise, 25 points for food and drink choices, and 25 for eating behavior for a "perfect" total of 100 points. Your goal is to score 100 points each day if possible. It may take several weeks or even a month or two to approach a perfect score, especially in the exercise area because of the need to begin and progress slowly. However, the higher you score, the more quickly you will reset the weight-regulating mechanism. So it is important to score as many points as you can right from the outset.

Figure 4.1

PROGRESS SUMMARY

Month	Day
EXERCISE	Poss
First 30 min. (½ pt./min.)	15
31 to 60 min. (1 pt./min.)	30
Correct Rate	5
Subtotal	50
FOOD & DRINK CHOICES	
1. Refined Carbohydrates	10
2. Fat Intake	10
3. Water Drinking	5
Subtotal	25
EATING BEHAVIOR	
4. End Main Meal Hunger	10
5. Meal Frequency	5
6. No Hunger Snacking	5
7. Faulty Drinking	5
Subtotal	25
TOTAL	100

SCORING TABLES

Food and Drink Choices

1. Refined Carbohydrates: Look up RCU's and allocate points as follows:

Total RCU	Pts.
0-2	10
3-4	8
5-6	6
7-8	4
9-10	2
11 or more	0

2. Fat Intake: Look up FU in table and allocate points as follows: Ideal Weight

Under 140 lbs.	Over 140 lbs	Pts.
0-4	0-5	10
5	6	7
6	7	3
7 +	8 +	0

3. Water Drinking:

	Pts.
6 glasses or more	5
5	4
4	3
3	2
2	1

Eating Behavior

4. End Main Meal Hunger

	Pts.
Complete satiety	10
No hunger, not satisfied	8
Slightly overfull or slightly hungry	5
Definitely overfull or def. hungry	0

5. Meal Frequency

	Pts.
3 or more	5
2	3
1	0

6. Times Snacking With No Hunger

	Pts.
0	5
1	4
2	3
3	2
4 or more	1

7. Faulty Drinking: 1 DU for any drink except water or skim milk.

DU	Pts.
0-1	5
2	4
3	2
4 or more	0

Figure 4.2 shows the other form used in the scoring system. This "daily record" form should be carried with you in your wallet or purse so you can record the amount and type of food you eat, your hunger level when you eat it, how much water you drink, and how long you exercise each day. The information you record on the daily record is scored and recorded on the progress summary each day. Blank daily record forms and progress summary forms are found at the back of the book and should be clipped out and used until you get a feel for the new lifestyle. We realize that we promised that there would be no "Mickey Mouse" requirements with this program. However, you must understand that the scoring system is entirely optional; if used, it needs be used only until you get a "feel" for the lifestyle change and can follow the principles on your own.

Figure 4.2   Daily Record

Date _____

Day	Meal	Time	Amount	Item	RCU	FU	DU	H
Exercise				Water	Total			

Meal: **B** = breakfast, **L** = light meal, **M** = main meal, **S** = snack.
H = hunger. Put an X for no hunger prior to snack

End of Main Meal Hunger/Satiety	**Points**
Completely satisfied	10
No hunger, but not completely satisfied	8
Slightly overfull or mild hunger	5
Definately overfull or moderate hunger	0

Recording Activity

First look at the daily record sheet that was filled out by an example patient (figure 4.3). He has recorded all three meals and a midafternoon snack. The "L" in the meal column at 7:30 a.m. and 12:30 p.m. refers to a "light" meal as discussed in chapter 3. The "M" refers to the "main" meal and the "S" indicates a snack as discussed in that same chapter. The only other food-related entry on the daily record is the "10" in the "H" or hunger column. This means that our patient was "completely satisfied" after eating the main meal (see the scoring guideline near the bottom of this form).

Figure 4.3   Daily Record

Date _____

Day	Meal	Time	Amount	Item	RCU	FU	DU	H
	L	7:30	1 c	skim milk				
			1 bowl	grapenuts				
			1 med.	grapefruit				
			1 sl.	whole wheat bread				
	L	12:30	1 bowl	tomato soup				
			1 sm	lettuce salad				
			1 diet	rootbeer				
	S	3:10	1 med.	apple				
	M	6:30	4 oz.	hamburger				10
		P	1 med.	baked potato				
			1 cup	carrots.				
			1 glass	skim milk				
			1 cup	jello				

Exercise **35 min**   Water **IN**   Total

Meal:**B** = breakfast, **L** = light meal, **M** = main meal, **S** = snack.
H = hunger. Put an X for no hunger prior to snack

End of Main Meal Hunger/Satiety	Points
Completely satisfied	10
No hunger, but not completely satisfied	8
Slightly overfull or mild hunger	5
Definately overfull or moderate hunger	0

It is helpful to evaluate hunger and satiety levels after each meal to achieve mastery of the eating drives. However, since it would likely be too cumbersome to do this for all meals, only main meal satiety is scored. Remember that for light meals you are to stop eating before feeling completely satisfied (see chapter 3 if you need to review this idea). However, eating to complete satiety once each day during the main meal will help avoid the starvation defenses as well as provide adequate vitamins and minerals. If you don't eat enough to satisfy your needs, you may be tempted to eat less desirable food later.

In the exercise block (bottom left) our patient recorded 35 minutes of exercise. He also recorded five glasses of water.

Scoring

The first major area to score is exercise. Only aerobic-type exercises that are steady and will keep the heart rate at the appropriate level qualify for points. Since the "Endurance Athlete Effect" is your goal, note on the progress summary under exercise (figure 4.4), that longer duration activity produces more points per minute. Five points are awarded if your heart rate reaches and maintains the appropriate level for your age and activity for most of the exercise period (see chapter 2 for heart rate guidelines).

Figure 4.4   PROGRESS SUMMARY

Month	Day													
EXERCISE	Poss													
First 30 min. (½ pt./min.)	15	15												
31 to 60 min. (1 pt./min.)	30	5												
Correct Rate	5	5												
Subtotal	50	25												

Our example patient exercised continuously for 35 minutes, so he received 15 points for the first 30 minutes (1/2 point per minute), five points for the five minutes after that (1 point per minute after 30 minutes), and five more points because he worked at the proper intensity for a total of 25 points (figure 4.4).

Although maximum points can be obtained by exercising for three different 30-minute periods during the day, it would be easier and usually more effective to do all your aerobic exercise at one time for a one-hour period.

We realize that this will be the most difficult guideline to follow. No one has a "free" hour to devote to exercise with the time demands of modern living. However, there is no other permanent way to achieve your goals. You must exercise faithfully if you expect results, especially if you have a long-term weight problem. After the setpoint is lowered, you may be able to decrease the duration and the frequency of exercise. Until then, exercise an hour a day, every day.

Food and Drink Choices

Twenty-five points are awarded for appropriate food and drink choices. Because you need to avoid refined carbohydrates and fats, we have developed a way to evaluate foods based on the amount of each contained in them. These values are expressed as refined carbohydrate units (RCU) or fat units (FU). The food tables that contain this information are found in appendix 13. An example from those tables is found below:

Item	Portion	RCU	FU	Cal	RCal	%Ft	P	F	C	Na
Taco Time:										
Burrito, meat	1	2	2	291		43	20	14	23	848
Burrito, soft bean	1	2	2	314		37	13	13	37	762
Taco	1	0	1	195		42	14	9	14	591
Soft Flour Taco	1	1	2	295		43	19	20	24	686
Supreme	1	1	3	356		51	19	20	24	696
Tangerine	1 med.	0	0	40	46	4	1	T	10	2

You can see that the meat burrito in the example contains both refined carbohydrate (2 RCU) and fat (2 FU). You will need to record the RCU and FU for each food on your daily record. It may be helpful at this point to practice scoring the main meal choices of our example patient. Look at the example below (figure 4.5). We have included the page number in the food table on which each item is found to

Figure 4.5

M	6:30 P	4oz.	hamburger	p. 188			
		1 med.	baked potato	p. 202			
		1 cup	carrots	p. 191			
		1 glass	skim milk	p. 199			
		1 cup	jello	p. 197			

Exercise **35 min.**   Water **IIII**   Total

help you find the FU and RCU for this practice problem. Before proceeding, turn to the food tables and score each entry for RCU and FU and record these values in the proper column.

Now that you have recorded the RCU and FU, check your answers with the example below. You should have scored two FU for the hamburger, nothing for potatoes, nothing for carrots and nothing for whole wheat bread or skim milk. One cup of Jell-O contains six RCU (three per 1/2 cup), so totals are: RCU six and FU two.

Figure 4.6   Daily Record

Date _____

Day	Meal	Time	Amount	Item	RCU	FU	DU	H
	L	7:30 A	1 cup	skim milk				
			1 bowl	grapenut flakes				
			1 med	grapefruit				
			1 sl.	whole wheat bread				
	L	12:30	1 bowl	tomato soup				
			1 med.	lettuce salad				
			1 diet	root beer				
	S	3:00	1 med	apple				
	M	6:30 P	4 oz.	hamburger		2		
			1 med	baked potato				
			1 serving	carrots				
			1 sl	whole wheat bread				
			8 oz.	skim milk				
			1 cup	jello	6			
Exercise **55 min.**				Water ┌┴┘	Total			

Now compute the number of points for RCU using "scoring table 1" on the example "progress summary" sheet below. In our example, six RCU were eaten so six points are recorded on the progress summary sheet on the refined carbohydrate line (figure 4.7).

Figure 4.7

FOOD & DRINK CHOICES							
1. Refined Carbohydrates	10	6					
2. Fat Intake	10						
3. Water Drinking	5						
Subtotal	25						

Food and Drink Choices
1. Refined Carbohydrates: Look up RCU's and allocate points as follows:

Total RCU	Pts.
0-2	10
3-4	8
5-6	6
7-8	4
9-10	2
11 or more	0

The amount of fat that is suitable depends on the "ideal" size of your body (you will make this computation in chapter 5). Our example patient's ideal weight is over 145 so he can consume up to five fat units and receive full points (see scoring table 2 in figure 4.8). Since our example diet contained only two FU, 10 points are scored and recorded on the progress summary sheet on the fat intake line.

Figure 4.8
PROGRESS SUMMARY

Month	Day															
EXERCISE	Poss															
First 30 min. (½ pt./min.)	15	15														
31 to 60 min. (1 pt./min.)	30	5														
Correct Rate	5	5														
Subtotal	50	25														
FOOD & DRINK CHOICES																
1. Refined Carbohydrates	10	6														
2. Fat Intake	10	10														
3. Water Drinking	5															
Subtotal	25															
EATING BEHAVIOR																
4. End Main Meal Hunger	10															
5. Meal Frequency	5															
6. No Hunger Snacking	5															
7. Faulty Drinking	5															
Subtotal	25															
TOTAL	100															

Food and Drink Choices   **SCORING TABLES**

1. Refined Carbohydrates: Look up RCU's and allocate points as follows:

Total RCU	Pts.
0-2	10
3-4	8
5-6	6
7-8	4
9-10	2
11 or more	0

2. Fat Intake: Look up FU in table and allocate points as follows:
Ideal Weight

Under 140 lbs.	Over 140 lbs	Pts.
0-4	0-5	10
5	6	7
6	7	3
7+	8+	0

3. Water Drinking

6 glasses or	5
	4
	3
	2

Water drinking. You should drink plenty of water, at least six glasses daily, but usually no more than 20 glasses. While you may add a drop or two of lemon juice, only plain water qualifies. Since our example patient drank five glasses of water, he would score and record four points on the progress summary (see scoring table 3, figure 4.9).

The "Food and Drink Choice" portion of the progress summary for our patient now shows 6 points for refined carbohydrates, 10 points for fat intake, and four points for water drinking for a total of 20 points (figure 4.9).

Figure 4.9 PROGRESS SUMMARY

Month	Day														
EXERCISE	Poss														
First 30 min. (½ pt./min.)	15														
31 to 60 min. (1 pt./min.)	30														
Correct Rate	5														
Subtotal	50														
FOOD & DRINK CHOICES															
1. Refined Carbohydrates	10	6													
2. Fat Intake	10	10													
3. Water Drinking	5	4													
Subtotal	25	20													

SCORING TABLES

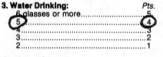

3. Water Drinking: Pts.
    6 glasses or more..........................5
    5...4
    4...3
    3...2
    2...1

Eating Behavior

The first factor under eating behavior relates to main meal hunger and has already been scored. The scoring table for this factor is on both the progress summary sheet (scoring table 4) and the daily record (near the bottom) because it needs to be evaluated just as you complete the main meal. Our example patient ate to complete satiety and scored 10 points on his daily summary immediately after he ate (see figure 4.10).

Meal frequency. The degree of hunger prior to mealtime is relatively unimportant since you should eat regularly even though not particularly hungry. Therefore, you get five points if you eat at least three times a day. Since our example patient ate three meals, he scored a full five points on the progress summary (see scoring table 5, figure 4.10).

Figure 4.10

EATING BEHAVIOR														
4. End Main Meal Hunger	10	*10*												
5. Meal Frequency	5	*5*												
6. No Hunger Snacking	5	*5*												
7. Faulty Drinking	5													
Subtotal	25													
TOTAL	**100**													

Eating Behavior

4. End Main Meal Hunger   *Pts.*
Complete satiety............................(10)
No hunger, not satisfied.......................8
Slightly overfull
   or slightly hungry.........................5
Definitely overfull
   or def. hungry.............................0

5. Meal Frequency   *Pts.*
3 or more...............................(5)
2..3
1..0

No-hunger snacking. The degree of hunger before a snack is very important and is scored, since snacking when no hunger is present causes more calories to be consumed than requested and you may not be able to waste them. If you snack when you are not hungry, you should place an "X" in the "H" column on the daily record. Enter scoring table 6 on the progress summary to determine the number of points in this area (figure 4.11). Our example patient snacked once, but was hungry so scored full points in this category. Try drinking a glass of water for a snack whenever you are hungry in case the feeling you have is really thirst.

Figure 4.11

6. Times Snacking With No Hunger   *Pts.*
0..(5)
1..4
2..3
3..2
4 or more....................................1

Faulty drinking. Most commonly used drinks either contain refined carbohydrates (sugar, alcohol) which are absorbed quickly; caffeine which stimulates insulin release; or artificial sweeteners, which contain sodium, raise your setpoint, and enhance your taste for sweets. All of these drinks cause problems for a person trying to control weight and should be replaced with water as soon as possible. We allow all the water you want to drink and two glasses of skim or 1 percent milk without losing points for improper drinking. Some drinks are worse than others. The list below shows how some of the most common drinks relate in terms of their effect on the setpoint (figure 4.12). This list is too long to be included on the progress summary, so you need to check it from time to time until you are familiar with the serving size that counts as one point. It would be best to avoid all these types of drinks, at least for the first few weeks. Note also that some drinks count in other scoring categories as well. For instance, a regular root beer contains seven RCU as well as a DU and whole milk contains one FU per cup.

Figure 4.12

Drink	Amount	DU
Soda pop with caffeine	6 oz.	1
Juice, soda pop, milk or beer	12 oz.	1
Wine	4 oz.	1
Distilled alcohol	2 oz.	1
Mixed drink	1 drink	1
Coffee/tea with cream and/or sugar	1 cup	1
Black coffee or tea	2 cups	1
Decaffeinated coffee w/cream & sugar	2 cups	1
Decaffeinated coffee, black	3 cups	1
Diet soda pop with caffeine	12 oz.	1
Diet soda pop, no caffeine	24 oz.	1
Skim or 1% milk (over 2 allowed glasses)	12 oz.	1

Our example patient drank one diet root beer and an "extra" glass of skim milk for a total of two drinking units (DU). Two DU yields four points for the faulty drinking category (see scoring table 7, figure 4.13) and the eating behavior category receives 24 out of the 25 possible points.

Figure 4.13

7. Faulty Drinking: 1 DU for any drink
except water or skim milk.

DU	Pts.
0-1	5
2	4
3	2
4 or more	0

Now turn to figure 4.14. This is the final progress summary form for our example patient. He received 25 out of 50 points for exercise, 20 out of 25 for food and drink choices, and 24 out of 25 in eating behavior for a total of 69 out of a possible 100 points. By analyzing this sheet, it is easy to see where improvement could be made. For instance, an apple instead of the Jell-O could have increased the

Figure 4.14

PROGRESS SUMMARY

Month	Day												
EXERCISE	Poss												
First 30 min. (½ pt./min.)	15	15											
31 to 60 min. (1 pt./min.)	30	15											
Correct Rate	5	5											
Subtotal	50	25											
FOOD & DRINK CHOICES													
1. Refined Carbohydrates	10	6											
2. Fat Intake	10	10											
3. Water Drinking	5	4											
Subtotal	25	20											
EATING BEHAVIOR													
4. End Main Meal Hunger	10	10											
5. Meal Frequency	5	5											
6. No Hunger Snacking	5	5											
7. Faulty Drinking	5	4											
Subtotal	25	24											
TOTAL	100	69											

SCORING TABLES

Food and Drink Choices

1. Refined Carbohydrates: Look up RCU's and allocate points as follows:

Total RCU	Pts.
0-2	10
3-4	8
5-6	6
7-8	4
9-10	2
11 or more	0

2. Fat Intake: Look up FU in table and allocate points as follows:

Ideal Weight		
Under 140 lbs.	Over 140 lbs	Pts.
0-4	0-5	10
5	6	7
6	7	3
7+	8+	0

3. Water Drinking:

	Pts.
6 glasses or more	5
5	4
4	3
3	2
2	1

Eating Behavior

4. End Main Meal Hunger | Pts.

	Pts.
Complete satiety	10
No hunger, not satisfied	8
Slightly overfull or slightly hungry	5
Definitely overfull or def. hungry	0

5. Meal Frequency | Pts.

	Pts.
3 or more	5
2	3
1	0

6. Times Snacking With No Hunger | Pts.

	Pts.
0	5
1	4
2	3
3	1
4 or more	0

7. Faulty Drinking: 1 DU for any drink except water or skim milk.

DU	Pts.
0-1	5
2	4
3	2
4 or more	0

score by four points and just 20 minutes more of exercise would have increased the total by 20 points. This extra 24 points could turn a rather mundane score of 69 into a blockbuster of 93.

You should use your progress summary to help you evaluate your progress just as our example patient used his. You may not score as many points initially as our example patient because you will not be as familiar with the types of food that contain refined carbohydrates and fat. However, as you score your daily record entries, you will soon memorize the unit values of many of the foods you eat, and you will make better choices as you score those that cause problems. You will also become aware of the other factors that are important for successful weight control. This system may seem difficult to use, but will be well worth the extra effort the first few weeks. After that you may wish to score yourself only occasionally to see how closely you are following the program. You may also find it useful to score yourself during problem times such as holidays and vacations. Keep in mind that the idea is to learn the principles and to make appropriate changes; there is no merit in padding points.

Although the number of points you score will be an excellent indicator of how well you are following the principles, there are other, less obvious indicators of success.

Other Indicators of Success

Most people use weight loss as the major indicator of success with dieting. The more weight they lose and the faster they lose it, the better they think they are doing. For some people, the tone of the entire day is determined by how much weight is lost or gained. The truth is that weight loss is really a very poor indicator of success. Body weight is a complex total of all the water, muscle, fat, and bones in your body. It varies from day to day and can be manipulated easily with no fat loss occurring. Using this program, you may lose weight rather slowly at first but still be losing fat very effectively. The following changes will help you realize you are making progress.

Measurements. As you lose fat, your waist, hips, thighs, and arm measurements will go down even if total body weight doesn't change. Measure several areas of your body and repeat these measurements every month or so.

How Clothes Fit. This may be the first indication that fat is being lost. If you have a pair of denim blue jeans that are really tight, you can use them as a fat-loss indicator. Try them on and evaluate how they fit. Put them away and don't wash or wear them. Try them on every few weeks and compare the fit to the previous trial. This may show a real change in your body when you might otherwise be discouraged by the scales.

How You Feel. When asked how they are doing, most people who have been on this program for a month or more will respond with something like, "I feel fantastic," or "I've never felt better." Most patients begin to feel better about themselves. They have more self-esteem, and feel less guilt. They usually become less judgemental about themselves and others. They accept themselves as being "okay" even if they are still fatter than they would like to be.

This "great" feeling is much more than the usual psychological initial boost from dieting; it is partly from living in harmony with the eating drives of the body, partly from eating adequate calories, vitamins and minerals, and partly from the far-reaching hormonal, enzymatic and metabolic changes which seem to occur with reprogramming. Whatever the cause, this is the part of our new program about which we are the most excited.

Energy Level. Almost everyone reports having more energy. Although some improvement occurs in a few days, most comes gradually as you improve your level of fitness and make other changes. The improvement in energy after several months is usually dramatic.

However, if you have been using heavy doses of caffeine or eating large quantities of refined carbohydrates, you may actually experience a type of "withdrawal" syndrome and may feel more tired for a period of time. If that occurs, stick with the program and the energy level will soon improve.

Improvements in Specific Health Problems. Many of our patients improve dramatically in overall health. They have fewer headaches, less constipation, and less nausea and indigestion. You may have a similar experience. In fact, if you are on medication for blood pressure or diabetes, you may need to be checked by your doctor fairly often because improvements in these conditions almost always occur, and medication may need to be decreased. Medications for headaches, arthritis, ulcers, anxiety, depression and sleep disturbances may also be reduced or eliminated (of course with your doctor's supervision).

Exercise. Our patients begin to enjoy exercise for the first time. They feel good both before and after they exercise. As they develop a regular pattern of exercise, they become more fit. They walk farther and faster and climb stairs with less puffing. If they haven't exercised, they miss it. Their body begins to perform as it was designed to perform.

Eating Control. Most of our patients develop a better relationship with food. They think about it less, have fewer cravings, and binge less often. They begin to be able to stop eating when they are full even if there is more food on the plate. They use food less for non-hunger needs and get into harmony with their hunger drives.

Healthier Foods. Most people begin to make better food choices. They find it easier to stay away from sugar and develop a taste for unsweetened food. They begin to learn more about foods. They read labels and evaluate other food they buy. They are able to eat bread and potatoes without guilt and learn to enjoy bread and vegetables with little or no butter.

Staying Encouraged

It might be helpful to write down how you feel in relation to the areas discussed above so that you can appreciate the changes that will occur in your life. Most people are amazed at how differently they feel in a few months, often finding it hard to believe that they ever felt as bad as their pre-program journal indicates. When you get discouraged and think you are not doing as well as you would like, read how you felt before starting the program. This should really make you aware of the many positive changes that are occurring.

Chapter Five
The New You

Now that you have learned how to exercise and eat to lower the weight setpoint, it is important to discuss what the body might look like when the setpoint has gone down. You need to realize that there is wide variability among people in the physical aspects of the body: height, weight, muscle mass, fat content, and body build.

Most of you have a preconceived idea of what your bodies should look like on the basis of the "ideal" body seen on TV, in movies, and in magazines. This idealized perception of what your body should look like is often much different from the real you. This is especially true for women whose perceptions of ideal body build are often based upon the ultrathin female fashion model.

For most women, these standards are unrealistic and perhaps unobtainable. Others may temporarily obtain them only through extreme starvation techniques that may trigger many serious health problems. In this chapter we will establish realistic weight goals so that you can enjoy your body at the weight it should really be.

The question then is how can realistic body weight goals be established? The "Gold Standard" of the past has been the Metropolitan Life Insurance tables for small-, medium-, and large-framed people. These tables were established by measuring large groups of people and using distribution curves to establish normality. Although quite accurate for many people, there are large discrepancies for others.

A much better way to determine proper body weight is to determine how much lean body mass (the entire body without any fat) a person has and then calculate the ideal body weight on the basis of that measurement. There are several ways to find lean body mass. All involve assessing body fat and calculating the lean body mass. For instance, some hospital and research centers use isotope studies or body water measurements. Fitness clinics and university research centers use hydrostatic weighing or skinfold techniques. In this chapter we have included charts that allow you to measure your percent body fat and then calculate the lean body mass using simple circumference measurements.

Being able to assess body composition is extremely useful. For example, men with muscular builds are often excluded from military service or from police forces because they weigh more than the height-weight charts permit. In many cases these men are not overfat at all; in fact, they may have less than average levels of fat. Their large bones, wide frames, and heavy muscles put them above the ideal levels on the height-weight charts, even though they are quite lean. For example, we hydrostatically weighed a 5' 9" football player who weighed 262 pounds but was only 12 percent fat.

The same problem exists with women. The height-weight charts are a poor guideline and can lead to mistaken ideas about ideal weight. The "eyeball" test is not very reliable either. Many women who look "fat" are in fact lean. Some who appear thin have a relatively high fat content. Since fat is only one of several major components of body shape, it is easy to see why these mistakes can be made. For example, several months ago, a young female athlete came into the office with her roommate. She wanted to lose weight and look more like her lighter, more feminine-looking friend.

The young athlete weighed 147 pounds and her roommate weighed only 115 pounds, even though both were nearly the same height. Of course, the athlete felt that she was overweight. Both girls were weighed underwater to determine the amount of fat on their bodies. Interestingly, the young athlete was only 14 percent fat while her roommate was nearly 22 percent fat. We have also weighed a 110 pound lady who was 40 percent fat. Obviously, total body weight has little to do with how fat you are.

Because of this wide individual variation in body type and build, the best way to determine a realistic weight goal is to measure how much fat you have, and from that information calculate a realistic weight based upon individual body type and build.

If you have inherited a mesomorphic or muscular body, you should weigh more than if you have inherited an ectomorphic or slender body because the basic nonfat portion of the body—the lean body mass—will be larger. In the case of the girl athlete and her roommate, the lean body mass (LBM) of the athlete was about 126 pounds, which is greater than the total body weight of her room-mate, even with no fat on her body.

The healthy amount of fat you should have is also variable. Young college-age men and women are normally leaner, that is, have less fat than older men and women. Women are also naturally fatter than men, due to the female hormones that direct extra fat to the hips and breasts. A realistic goal in terms of body fat is shown in figure 5.1. Note that there is a wide range of fat that is considered "normal." You shouldn't be concerned if you are within this range, whether on the high or low end.

Figure 5.1

Ideal percent fat goals for men and women

	Men	Women
% Fat	15 - 22%	20% - 28%

We have included some tables to help you determine your current percent body fat using simple circumference measurements. These tests are not as accurate as hydrostatic weighing, but they are a good estimate for people who do not have access to hydrostatic tanks and will be valuable in helping determine the basic Lean Body Mass (LBM) so you can compute the most realistic total weight.

Use the applicable section below to predict the percent fat.

Predicting Body Fat for Women

To get a good estimate of the percentage of body fat, you should measure the following areas with a cloth tape measure. Pull the tape lightly but firmly around the areas to be measured and measure over bare skin if possible. You should be sure to keep the tape level during the measurement and take two or three measurements each of the following sites to get a good average:

- Hips - measure around the hips at the maximum girth.
- Abdomen - measure around the waist at the umbilicus (belly button).
- Measure the height in inches.

Computation Form

Hips Average
Measurement _____   Constant A _____
                                           (from Table 5-1)

Abdomen Average
Measurement _____   Constant B _____ add A & B _____
Height in inches _____   Constant C _____ minus C _____
                            Equals % Fat _____

Put the average of your measurements in the blank space on the
computation form. Now look at the "hips" column in table 5.1. Note
that there is a number to the right side of each hip measurement.
This number is a "constant" and is used in the computation of percent body fat from the measurements you have taken. Write down
the constant for each measurement you have made on the computation form to the right side of the measurement. Now add constant A
to constant B and subtract constant C. The number you have left is
percent body fat.

An example may be helpful. If a lady had an average hip circumference of 42 inches and an average abdominal circumference of
28 and was 64 inches tall, we would get the following calculations:

Hips Average
Measurement:_____42____   Constant A_____50.24_____
Abdominal Average
Measurement_____28____   Constant B__19.91__Add A & B 70.15
Height inches:_____64____   Constant C___39.00__Minus C 39.00
                            Equals % Fat_31.15_____

According to these measurements, she is about 31 percent fat.

Predicting Body Fat for Men

It is quite easy to get percent fat for men since only the wrist and
waist are measured. First, measure your waist at the umbilical (belly
button) and then have someone measure your wrist circumference
just in front of the wrist bones where the wrist bends. Now subtract
the wrist measurement from the waist measurement and enter the
chart with this number and your weight.

For example, if your waist is 34 inches, and your wrist is 7 inches,
the difference is 27 (34 − 7 = 27). If you weigh 175 lbs., go down the
"27" column to 175 and read 15 percent fat.

Table 5.1. Conversion Constants to Predict Percent Body Fat (Women)

	Hips		Abdomen		Height
In.	Constant A	In.	Constant B	In.	Constant C
30	33.48	20	14.22	55	33.52
31	34.87	21	14.93	56	34.13
32	36.27	22	15.64	57	34.74
33	37.67	23	16.35	58	35.35
34	39.06	24	17.06	59	35.96
35	40.46	25	17.78	60	36.57
36	41.86	26	18.49	61	37.18
37	43.25	27	19.20	62	37.79
38	44.65	28	19.91	63	38.40
39	46.05	29	20.62	64	39.01
40	47.44	30	21.33	65	39.62
41	48.84	31	22.04	66	40.23
42	50.24	32	22.75	67	40.84
43	51.64	33	23.46	68	41.45
44	53.03	34	24.18	69	42.06
45	54.43	35	24.89	70	42.67
46	55.83	36	25.60	71	43.28
47	57.22	37	26.31	72	43.89
48	58.62	38	27.02	73	44.50
49	60.02	39	27.73	74	45.11
50	61.42	40	28.44	75	45.72
51	62.81	41	29.15	76	46.32
52	64.21	42	29.87	77	46.93
53	65.61	43	30.58	78	47.54
54	67.00	44	31.29	79	48.15
55	68.40	45	32.00	80	48.76
56	69.80	46	32.71	81	49.37
57	71.19	47	33.42	82	49.98
58	72.59	48	34.13	83	50.59
59	73.99	49	34.84	84	51.20
60	75.39	50	35.56	85	51.81

From The Complete Book of Physical Fitness, A.G. Fisher and R.K. Conlee, used by permission.

BODY FAT PERCENTAGES FROM THE PENROSE–NELSON–FISHER EQUATIONS
WAIST MINUS WRIST (INCHES)

WT (LBS)	22	22.5	23	23.5	24	24.5	25	25.5	26	26.5	27	27.5	28	28.5
120	4	6	8	10	12	14	16	18	20	21	23	25	27	29
125	4	6	7	9	11	13	15	17	19	20	22	24	26	28
130	3	5	7	9	11	12	14	16	18	20	21	23	25	27
135	3	5	7	8	10	12	13	15	17	19	20	22	24	26
140	3	5	6	8	10	11	13	15	16	18	19	21	23	24
145	3	4	6	7	9	11	12	14	15	17	19	20	22	23
150	2	4	6	7	9	10	12	13	15	16	18	19	21	23
155	2	4	5	7	8	10	11	13	14	16	17	19	20	22
160	2	4	5	6	8	9	11	12	14	15	17	18	19	21
165	2	3	5	6	8	9	10	12	13	15	16	17	19	20
170	2	3	4	6	7	9	10	11	13	14	15	17	18	19
175	2	3	4	6	7	8	10	11	12	13	15	16	17	19
180	1	3	4	5	7	8	9	10	12	13	14	16	17	18
185	1	3	4	5	6	8	9	10	11	13	14	15	16	18
190	1	2	4	5	6	7	8	10	11	12	13	15	16	17
195	1	2	3	5	6	7	8	9	11	12	13	14	15	16
200	1	2	3	4	6	7	8	9	10	11	12	14	15	16
205	1	2	3	4	5	6	8	9	10	11	12	13	14	15
210	1	2	3	4	5	6	7	8	9	11	12	13	14	15
215	1	2	3	4	5	6	7	8	9	10	11	12	13	15
220	0	2	3	4	5	6	7	8	9	10	11	12	13	14
225	0	1	2	3	4	6	7	8	9	10	11	12	13	14
230	0	1	2	3	4	5	6	7	8	9	10	11	12	13
235	0	1	2	3	4	5	6	7	8	9	10	11	12	13
240	0	1	2	3	4	5	6	7	8	9	10	11	12	13
245	0	1	2	3	4	5	6	7	8	9	9	10	11	12
250	0	1	2	3	4	5	6	6	7	8	9	10	11	12
255	0	1	2	3	3	4	5	6	7	8	9	10	11	12
260	0	1	2	2	3	4	5	6	7	8	9	10	10	11
265	0	1	1	2	3	4	5	6	7	8	8	9	10	11
270	0	1	1	2	3	4	5	6	7	7	8	9	10	11
275	0	0	1	2	3	4	5	5	6	7	8	9	10	11
280	0	0	1	2	3	4	4	5	6	7	8	9	9	10
285	0	0	1	2	3	4	4	5	6	7	8	8	9	10
290	0	0	1	2	3	3	4	5	6	7	7	8	9	10
295	0	0	1	2	2	3	4	5	6	6	7	8	9	10
300	0	0	1	2	2	3	4	5	5	6	7	8	9	9

Penrose, Nelson and Fisher, "Generalized Body Composition Prediction Equation for Men Using Simple Measurement Techniques. <u>Medicine and Science in Sports and Exercise</u> Vol. 17, No. 2, April, 1985.

29	29.5	30	30.5	31	31.5	32	32.5	33	33.5	34	34.5	35	35.5	36
31	33	35	37	39	41	43	45	47	49	50	52	54	56	58
30	32	33	35	37	39	41	43	45	46	48	50	52	54	56
28	30	32	34	36	37	39	41	43	44	46	48	50	52	53
27	29	31	32	34	36	38	39	41	43	44	46	48	50	51
26	28	29	31	33	34	36	38	39	41	43	44	46	48	49
25	27	28	30	31	33	35	36	38	39	41	43	44	46	47
24	26	27	29	30	32	33	35	36	38	40	41	43	44	46
23	25	26	28	29	31	32	34	35	37	38	40	41	43	44
22	24	25	27	28	30	31	33	34	35	37	38	40	41	43
22	23	24	26	27	29	30	31	33	34	36	37	38	40	41
21	22	24	25	26	28	29	30	32	33	34	36	37	39	40
20	21	23	24	25	27	28	29	31	32	33	35	36	37	39
19	21	22	23	25	26	27	28	30	31	32	34	35	36	37
19	20	21	23	24	25	26	28	29	30	31	33	34	35	36
18	19	21	22	23	24	26	27	28	29	30	32	33	34	35
18	19	20	21	22	24	25	26	27	28	30	31	32	33	34
17	18	19	21	22	23	24	25	26	28	29	30	31	32	33
17	18	19	20	21	22	23	25	26	27	28	29	30	31	32
16	17	18	19	21	22	23	24	25	26	27	28	29	30	32
16	17	18	19	20	21	22	23	24	25	26	28	29	30	31
15	16	17	18	19	20	22	23	24	25	26	27	28	29	30
15	16	17	18	19	20	21	22	23	24	25	26	27	28	29
14	15	16	17	18	19	20	21	22	23	24	25	26	27	28
14	15	16	17	18	19	20	21	22	23	24	25	26	27	28
14	15	16	17	17	18	19	20	21	22	23	24	25	26	27
13	14	15	16	17	18	19	20	21	22	23	24	25	26	27
13	14	15	16	17	18	18	19	20	21	22	23	24	25	26
13	14	14	15	16	17	18	19	20	21	22	23	24	24	25
12	13	14	15	16	17	18	19	19	20	21	22	23	24	24
12	13	14	15	15	16	17	18	19	20	21	22	22	23	24
12	13	13	14	15	16	17	18	19	19	20	21	22	23	24
11	12	13	14	15	16	16	17	18	19	20	21	22	22	23
11	12	13	14	14	15	16	17	18	19	19	20	21	22	23
11	12	12	13	14	15	16	17	17	18	19	20	21	21	22
11	11	12	13	14	15	15	16	17	18	19	19	20	21	22
10	11	12	13	14	14	15	16	17	17	18	19	20	21	21
10	11	12	12	13	14	15	16	16	17	18	19	19	20	21

BODY FAT PERCENTAGES FROM THE PENROSE-NELSON-FISHER EQUATIONS
WAIST MINUS WRIST (INCHES)

WT (LBS)	36.5	37	37.5	38	38.5	39	39.5	40	40.5	41	41.5	42	42.5	43
120	60	62	64	66	68	70	72	74	76	77	79	81	83	85
125	58	59	61	63	65	67	69	71	72	74	76	78	80	82
130	55	57	59	61	62	64	66	68	69	71	73	75	77	78
135	53	55	56	58	60	62	63	65	67	68	70	72	74	75
140	51	53	54	56	58	59	61	63	64	66	68	69	71	72
145	49	51	52	54	55	57	59	60	62	63	65	67	68	70
150	47	49	50	52	53	55	57	58	60	61	63	64	66	67
155	46	47	49	50	52	53	55	56	58	59	61	62	64	65
160	44	46	47	48	50	51	53	54	56	57	59	60	61	63
165	43	44	45	47	48	50	51	52	54	55	57	58	60	61
170	41	43	44	45	47	48	49	51	52	54	55	56	58	59
175	40	41	43	44	45	47	48	49	51	52	53	55	56	57
180	39	40	41	43	44	45	47	48	49	50	52	53	54	56
185	38	39	40	41	43	44	45	46	48	49	50	51	53	54
190	37	38	39	40	41	43	44	45	46	48	49	50	51	52
195	35	37	38	39	40	41	43	44	45	46	47	49	50	51
200	35	36	37	38	39	40	41	43	44	45	46	47	48	50
205	34	35	36	37	38	39	40	41	43	44	45	46	47	48
210	33	34	35	36	37	38	39	40	42	43	44	45	46	47
215	32	33	34	35	36	37	38	39	40	42	43	44	45	46
220	31	32	33	34	35	36	37	38	39	41	42	43	44	45
225	30	31	32	33	34	35	36	37	38	40	41	42	43	44
230	30	31	32	33	34	35	36	37	38	39	40	41	42	43
235	29	30	31	32	33	34	35	36	37	38	39	40	41	42
240	28	29	30	31	32	33	34	35	36	37	38	39	40	41
245	27	28	29	30	31	32	33	34	35	36	37	38	39	40
250	27	28	29	30	31	31	32	33	34	35	36	37	38	39
255	26	27	28	29	30	31	32	33	34	34	35	36	37	38
260	26	27	27	28	29	30	31	32	33	34	35	35	36	37
265	25	26	27	28	29	29	30	31	32	33	34	35	36	36
270	25	25	26	27	28	29	30	31	31	32	33	34	35	36
275	24	25	26	27	27	28	29	30	31	32	32	33	34	35
280	24	24	25	26	27	28	29	29	30	31	32	33	33	34
285	23	24	25	26	26	27	28	29	30	30	31	32	33	34
290	23	23	24	25	26	27	27	28	29	30	31	31	32	33
295	22	23	24	25	25	26	27	28	28	29	30	31	32	32
300	22	22	23	24	25	26	26	27	28	29	29	30	31	32

43.5	44	44.5	45	45.5	46	46.5	47	47.5	48	48.5	49	49.5	50
87	89	91	93	95	97	99	99	99	99	99	99	99	99
84	85	87	89	91	93	95	96	98	99	99	99	99	99
80	82	84	86	87	89	91	93	94	96	98	99	99	99
77	79	80	82	84	86	87	89	91	92	94	96	98	99
74	76	77	79	81	82	84	86	87	89	91	92	94	96
71	73	75	76	78	79	81	83	84	86	87	89	91	92
69	70	72	74	75	77	78	80	81	83	84	86	87	89
67	68	70	71	73	74	76	77	79	80	82	83	85	86
64	66	67	69	70	72	73	75	76	77	79	80	82	83
62	64	65	67	68	69	71	72	74	75	76	78	79	81
60	62	63	64	66	67	69	70	71	73	74	75	77	78
59	60	61	63	64	65	66	68	69	70	72	73	74	76
57	58	59	61	62	63	65	66	67	68	70	71	72	74
55	56	58	59	60	61	63	64	65	66	68	69	70	71
54	55	56	57	58	60	61	62	63	65	66	67	68	69
52	53	55	56	57	58	59	60	62	63	64	65	66	68
51	52	53	54	55	57	58	59	60	61	62	63	65	66
49	51	52	53	54	55	56	57	58	60	61	62	63	64
48	49	50	51	53	54	55	56	57	58	59	60	61	62
47	48	49	50	51	52	53	54	56	57	58	59	60	61
46	47	48	49	50	51	52	53	54	55	56	57	58	59
45	46	47	48	49	50	51	52	53	54	55	56	57	58
44	45	46	47	48	49	50	51	52	53	54	55	56	57
42	43	44	45	46	47	48	49	50	51	52	53	54	55
41	42	43	44	44	45	46	47	48	49	50	51	52	53
40	41	42	43	44	44	45	46	47	48	49	50	51	52
39	40	41	42	43	44	44	45	46	47	48	49	50	51
38	39	40	41	42	43	43	44	45	46	47	48	49	50
37	38	39	40	41	42	43	43	44	45	46	47	48	49
37	37	38	39	40	41	42	43	43	44	45	46	47	48
36	37	38	38	39	40	41	42	43	43	44	45	46	47
35	36	37	38	38	39	40	41	42	43	43	44	45	46
34	35	36	37	38	39	39	40	41	42	43	43	44	45
34	35	35	36	37	38	38	39	39	40	41	42	43	44
33	34	35	36	36	37	38	39	39	40	41	42	43	43
33	33	34	35	36	36	37	38	39	39	40	41	42	43

Record your waist measurement _____
Record your wrist measurement _____
Difference _____

Now enter the column in the table with this difference and go down to your weight.   _____

This number is your percent fat _____

Computing Lean Body Mass

Although it is interesting to see how much of the body is fat, you need to compute lean body mass (LBM) to compute a realistic body weight.

There are two steps that must be taken to compute lean body mass.

- Step one: Multiply the body weight in pounds by the percent fat. This will give pounds of fat on the body. For example, the lady in our example was 31 percent fat. If she weighed 160 pounds, she would have about 49.6 pounds of fat.

Total Weight x %Fat = lbs. of fat
160 x .31 (31%) = 49.6 lbs. of fat

- Step two: To determine the LBM, simply subtract pounds of fat from total body weight.

Total Weight — Pounds of Fat = LBM
160 lbs. total weight — 49.6 lbs. fat = 110.4 lbs. LBM

Anything that is not fat is lean, so the fat and lean components must add up to the total body weight.

This LBM is the "real" person without any fat. Obviously, you can't weigh less than your LBM, nor can you get along without any fat. All of us need at least some fat to support the internal organs and to give shape to our frame. The very leanest men sometimes get as low as 2 to 3 percent fat while the leanest women are from 9 to 11 percent fat.

Table 5.3 - Total body weight at various fat percentages
based on lean body mass

			% Fat Goal			
LBM	10	13	16	19	22	25
90	100	103	107	111	115	120
95	105	109	113	117	121	126
100	111	114	119	123	128	133
105	116	120	125	129	134	140
110	122	126	130	135	141	146
115	127	132	136	141	147	153
120	133	137	142	148	153	160
125	138	143	148	154	160	166
130	144	149	154	160	166	173
135	150	155	160	166	173	180
140	155	160	166	172	179	186
145	161	166	172	179	185	193
150	166	172	178	185	192	200
155	172	178	184	191	198	206
160	177	183	190	197	205	213
165	183	189	196	203	211	220
170	188	195	202	209	217	226
175	194	201	208	216	224	233
180	200	206	214	222	230	240
185	205	212	220	228	237	246

LBM in pounds (vertical axis label)

Computing a Realistic Weight Goal

To compute a realistic weight, you must decide what percent fat
you are willing to have. A realistic beginning goal for the woman in
our example may be 25 percent. Enter table 5.3 with the LBM and go
across to the percent fat goal to get a realistic weight goal. For our example lady, whose LBM is 110 pounds, the realistic weight would be
about 146 pounds.

This may be a higher weight than our example lady would care
to achieve, but it is realistic, and she would be about 25 percent fat if
she achieved that weight.

Another factor needs to be considered. Sometimes the LBM goes
up or down during the weight loss process. An extremely heavy person may have a larger LBM than usual because the muscle mass
hypertrophied (got larger) from carrying all the weight around.
When this person loses fat, he may also lose LBM because the load

on the muscles is decreased.

On the other hand, an inactive person may have a decreased LBM because he is so inactive. When this person begins an exercise program, he may experience a gain in LBM back to some normal level. This gain in lean tissue can be discouraging because it may counteract the loss of fat, and the total body weight may stay about the same or even increase, even though the person is losing fat nicely.

One patient maintained the same weight (330 pounds) for four weeks, even though he lost almost seven inches of waist measurement during that time. He was discouraged but continued his program and finally began to lose weight. You should not be discouraged if this happens to you. Remember, a slow, gradual loss is usually the type of loss associated with permanent, long-term change. Some of the advertised weight-loss programs (30 pounds a month) are unrealistic, unhealthful and never yield good long-term results. We are happiest with a one- to two- pound change a week.

You should check your hip and waist measurements each month to determine what is happening to LBM and percent fat. If the LBM changes, you can compute a new realistic weight goal based on this change. The measurements will also permit seeing the circumference changes as they occur.

Other Factors to Consider

Realistic weight will not necessarily be the weight dreamed of, nor will it necessarily be a weight that will permit looking like the models in the fashion magazines. In fact, you may be surprisingly close to a realistic body weight right now. If so, don't fight it—accept it and enjoy the feeling it gives.

One group of home-economics teachers computed their realistic body weights; nearly half were right where they should have been. Some of them had struggled for years to get to a lower weight and felt badly all that time because they weren't successful in reaching a lower weight.

Another factor involves the setpoint of the weight-regulating mechanism. We know that the principles in this book work to readjust the setpoint, but we are never really sure how far down it will go. Some people go to a lower level quite easily, but others will never reach their realistic weight goal. If you carefully follow the principles of diet and exercise and still do not reach your calculated realistic weight, you may have to accept a higher weight. If this is the case, you should be philosophical and accept the lowest weight you can reach. Rigid restrictions in intake or fad diets may decrease the weight for a short time, but these starvation techniques may actually adjust the setpoint higher and make the weight problem worse. In the long run you will level off at the setpoint the body chooses, and it will be the lowest it can be when you follow the principles in this book.

Understanding more about the basis of your weight, you should be able to feel better about yourself and enjoy life more. If you hate your body, thinking of yourself as being fat and ugly, and out of control, you will find it difficult to enjoy life. People who feel like this tend to put off enjoyment of life until they become thin. They say, "When I am thin I will be able to go swimming with my children" or, "When I am skinny I will take up skiing or tennis; when I am thin I will be more attractive to my husband; when I am thin I will be more outgoing and others will like me better; when I am thin all my problems will vanish." With this attitude, they usually never really enjoy life, since few become or stay as thin as they would like. Those who do lose weight often find they still feel the same way about themselves and their problems have not disappeared.

Most authorities agree that a healthy self-image helps to prevent physical and emotional problems. For many of you, developing a healthy self-image involves making changes in attitude about your body. Developing a realistic impression of what your body should look like and how much you should weigh will be very helpful in accepting yourself.

We wish you great success in your efforts to get in harmony with your body and lose weight to the point that your setpoint will accept realistically. We have been impressed with the success of many of our patients and know that you can be successful too.

A COMPARISON OF THE EFFECTS OF LOW CALORIE DIETS AND THE REPROGRAMMING PLAN

Measure	During Reducing Phase		Long-Term	
	Low Calorie	Reprogramming Plan	Low Calorie	Reprogramming Plan
Physical				
Body Weight Loss:				
First Few Weeks	+ Fast	– Slow or gain		
1-4 Months	– Slows Down	+ Speeds Up		
After 4 Months	– Stops	+ Moderate		
Body Weight	+ Decreases	+ Decreases	– Increases	+ Stable
Tendency to stay lighter			– Low	+ High
Body Fat	– Decreases	+ Decreases	– Increases	+ Stays Low
Muscle Tissue	– Decreases	+ Increases	– Moderate	+ High
Weight Set Point	– Same or Higher	+ Lower	– High	+ Low
Biochemical				
Body Sugar & Water Stores	– Decreases	+ Normalizes	– Low to Normal	+ Normal
Bone Density	– Decreases	+ Increases	– Low to Normal	+ High
Intestinal Contents	– Low	+ High Bulk	– Moderate	+ High Bulk
Metabolic Rate	– Decreases	+ High	– Low to Moderate	+ High
Fat Burning Enzymes	– Decreases	+ Increases	– Low	+ High
Insulin Resistance	+ Decreases	+ Decreases	– Normal or Higher	+ Lower
Energy Conservation	– Increases	+ Decreases	– High	+ Normal
Energy Wasting	– Decreases	+ Normal	– Low	+ Normal
Feelings				
Energy Level	– Decreases	+ Increases	– Low to Moderate	+ High
Strength	– Decreases	+ Increases	– Low to Moderate	+ High
Endurance	– Decreases	+ Increases	– Low to Moderate	+ High
Stress of Plan	– High	+ Moderate to Low	– Moderate to High	+ Low
Hunger	– High	+ Normal	– Moderate to High	+ Normal
Tendency to Binge	– High	+ Low	– High	+ Low
Sugar Cravings	– High	+ Low	– High	+ Low
Thinking About Food	– Constantly	+ Occasionally	– Moderate to High	+ Infrequent
Times When "Feeling Good"	– Low	+ High	– Low to Moderate	+ High
Self Esteem	+ High	+ High	– Low	+ High
Number of Positive or Helpful Effects (+)	5	24	0	23
Number of Negative or Harmful Effects (–)	20	1	23	0

Appendix One
Evidence for a Weight-Regulating Mechanism

We would now like to present some evidence that the WRM does exist and exerts a powerful influence, and that there is a strong tendency for the body to stabilize weight at a particular level and defend that weight.

Tendency to Maintain a Stable Body Weight

One of the standard questions on most medical forms for life insurance relates to significant weight loss or gain during the previous year. It is surprising how often an applicant responds that not only has the weight remained the same for the last year, but that it has remained stable for the past 10 to 20 years. One of the authors has probably eaten 32 million calories over the past 30 years and has gone through a wide variety of physical activity, yet weighs exactly what he weighed in high school. We all know people who weigh the same year after year and who make no attempt to control food intake nor activity level. Those whose weight has changed have usually been influenced by pregnancy or other factors which we will soon discuss that are known to change the setpoint of the WRM. There is a tendency to gain a few pounds every 10 years or so, but this gain is remarkably small in most cases. This small increase in weight usually reflects a minor adjustment in the setpoint of the WRM. When you understand the factors that control the WRM, you will understand why people sometimes experience an increase in weight. Your own observations of these factors in your own life or the life of a friend will provide evidence for the existence of the WRM.

Ineffectiveness of Dieting

If the body weight were not closely regulated, it would be much easier to lose and gain weight. If weight loss were merely a reflection of total caloric intake, it would be a simple matter to lose weight by simply missing breakfast and eating normally the rest of the day. Theoretically, this should result in a 30- to 50- pound loss each year. With more drastic changes in eating patterns, we would expect to see even more dramatic weight changes. For instance, a change from 3000 calories to 1000 calories daily would theoretically reduce weight by 17 pounds the first month, and by over 200 pounds in a year.

Although the predicted weight gains or losses may occur over a short period of time with altered food intake, they are seldom seen for long periods of time. After the initial loss (which may be as much muscle and water as fat), the body weight tends to stabilize at some new lower level and no further change occurs.

Some researchers have theorized that this failure to lose weight reflects the decreased energy need in the body which has been made smaller by the dieting process. Although our energy needs may fall a little, we should still be able to continue effective weight loss with a reduced calorie diet. Since we seldom see continuous weight loss at the predicted rate, there must be other influences involved. The major influence in preventing continued weight loss seems to be the WRM. Through its sensor systems, the WRM becomes "aware" that food intake is limited and that fat stores are becoming depleted. It "recognizes" this situation as dangerous, and directs changes in the body to conserve energy. The body can then function at a lower energy level, and weight loss stops or slows dramatically. The body is now much more efficient and can regain the lost fat with only a small increase in food intake. In addition, hunger is greatly increased, and the dieter becomes more and more driven by a powerful need to eat. This drive usually becomes so strong that few people can follow low calorie diets for long.

This mechanism explains the failure of traditional diets. Only about 25 percent of all dieters succeed in losing 20 pounds; and of those who need to lose more than 40 pounds, only 5 percent are able to do so.

An even more dramatic evidence of the WRM is the tendency of dieters to regain lost weight. More than 90 percent of them return to their previous weight within two years. It is interesting how often their weights are within a fraction of a pound of their previous weight. This is not only strong evidence of a regulating mechanism, but also evidence that it is sensitive to minor weight changes, and able to control the weight within a very narrow range.

Starvation Studies

Various animal and human volunteer starvation studies have shown evidence of a weight regulator, and insight into its actions. Animal studies (where food intake can be much more closely controlled) have shown that when a starving animal is again allowed to eat all it wants it will quickly gain back its previous weight. A growing rat who has been deprived of food will gain weight 20 times faster than its genetically identical litter mates when allowed to eat the same amount of food that they are eating, even though no extra food is given to compensate for the period of time that food was withheld. When they are provided all the food they want, the starved rats will eat more than their control littermates, and even more quickly gain weight to the expected level.

These studies provide clear evidence of a mechanism that closely controls weight by controlling energy balance and directing food intake. A notable human starvation study was done during World War II with a group of conscientious objectors. They were placed on a starvation diet consisting of one-half of their usual food intake. As time passed and they became progressively more hungry, food became the most important thing in their lives. They began to dream about food and think about it most of the time. They even planned career changes to become bakers, waiters in restaurants, or work in other food-related fields. They became fatigued, lethargic and apathetic, and much less active. The WRM seemed to direct them to eat, but decreased their activity level to conserve energy.

When the forced starvation period was ended and they were allowed to return to normal eating, they never felt satisfied. Even after a big meal, they felt a desire to eat more. This feeling did not leave until their weight had returned to its normal level. At this point, normal hunger drives returned and each subject returned to his normal eating and activity patterns.

Several observations related to this study suggest evidence of a WRM. The return to the previous stable weight is good evidence. The strong desire to eat even after eating a full meal suggests a driving mechanism designed to encourage enough eating to quickly regain the previous stable weight. The fatigue, apathy, and decreased activity during the starvation period suggest a mechanism designed to conserve energy and prevent further weight loss.

Liquid Formula Diets

An another interesting study was done wherein the total food intake for a group of volunteers was provided by a nutritious liquid obtained by sucking it from an unseen receptacle through a straw-like apparatus. Within a few days, subjects adjusted their intake to match their daily needs. When the caloric content of the liquid was doubled or halved (with no change in flavor or texture), the subjects would automatically decrease or increase their intake within a couple of days to supply the needed calories. At the end of the study, the weight of each subject had remained the same. This study again suggests evidence of an ability to measure and regulate food intake to maintain a constant body weight.

Force-Feeding Studies

Several force-feeding studies have been performed on both animals and humans. Similar results have been observed. In some people, even huge amounts of extra eating will fail to cause weight gain. These people seem to have a weight-regulating mechanism that can vigorously defend the selected weight by wasting huge quantities of excess energy intake.

Most force-fed subjects will gain only a limited amount of weight and will then gain no more, despite a continued excess of food. This gain suggests a regulating mechanism that stimulates the wasting of extra energy to maintain the weight at some set level. These energy wasting processes are probably present in most of us, but may never have been fully developed. Since most Americans eat more than the minimum required to stabilize weight, we must all be regularly wasting some energy.

Another facet of the force-feeding studies that points to a WRM is that most of these subjects will quickly return to the pre-study weight even though no continous effort is made to diet. The WRM will indefinitely prevent us from gaining weight, even on huge amounts of excess food, but seems more designed to protect us from undereating or starvation.

Case Study with Increased Intake

A German scientist carefully measured his caloric intake for one full year and noted that he ate an average of 1760 calories per day. During the next year, he increased his caloric intake by 400 calories daily. At the end of the year, he was still very close to his original weight even though he had eaten enough extra energy to have gained over 40 pounds. He then increased his intake another 600 calories a day for another year without changing his original weight. Theoretically, he should have gained 60 pounds the second year, making a total of more than 100 pounds that he should have gained over the two-year period. This study is evidence of a WRM that can control the body weight within certain limits despite varying food intake.

Brain Surgery

Rat studies have been done where part of the hypothalamus was destroyed. If the particular area that controls the feeding drive (the feeding center) is surgically damaged, the animal will eat very little and will dramatically decrease weight. If the part of the brain controlling satiety or satisfaction (the satiety center) is destroyed, then the animal will eat more than usual and gain weight. He will then stabilize at the higher level and defend that weight. Both of these animal models will respond in the same way as normal rats to exercise and dietary factors that change the weight. If activity level increases, all three groups will lose weight, and if activity is decreased, all three groups will gain weight. These lesions seem to change the level at which the WRM is set. It still defends the body weight as before, but now defends a different weight level.

Brain Damage

There have been case reports where the part of the human brain that influences eating has been damaged through accident or disease. In some of these cases, a feeling of fullness or satiety is never reached and continuous hunger encourages excessive eating. In these cases, weight gain continues to a very high level, sometimes until death occurs. This is unlike the force-feeding studies where continued excess food intake only produced modest weight gain. In these brain damage cases, the WRM no longer functions to provide for energy wasting. A comparison between these brain damages, malfunctioning cases, and "normal" people gives good evidence of a weight-regulating mechanism that directs appropriate food intake and energy balance.

Appendix Two
Regulation of Eating and the Insulin Mechanism

Food Intake Regulator. The food intake regulator has a very profound influence in our lives. Animal studies have shown hungry animals will undergo extreme discomfort, such as running across an electric grid, to reach food. Humans have also been known to risk death, serious injury or severe punishment to get food when they are hungry enough. In this chapter, we will outline a simplified model of the food intake regulator to help you understand the complexity and power of this mechanism.

The control center for eating is located in the hypothalamus, along with the weight-regulating mechanism. It consists of a feeding center which is activated when there is a need for food and a satiety center which is activated when we are full or satisfied by our intake of food. Information is provided from many different sources. For instance, the food is smelled and tasted and the amount of chewing and swallowing is sensed. Even stomach distention is measured by stretch receptors in the stomach wall. Messages from the stomach affect the satiety and feeding center directly by way of the vagus nerve (see Fig. A2.1).

In the intestines, digestive enzymes are released in response to various foods, and the amount of these enzymes affects the food intake regulators. The blood and tissue levels of the various foods are also sensed. If liver or blood sugar is low, or if fat cell size has changed, the body senses these changes and increases or decreases the appetite to compensate. An example may help you understand how these factors affect our hunger. If you needed 1,000 calories to meet your energy needs on any given day, you could ingest four ounces of vegetable oil or eat 20 pounds of lettuce. If you chose to use the vegetable oil, there would really be very little tasting, chewing, or swallowing and those four ounces would not begin to fill up the stomach. Although you would receive enough calories, you would probably still be hungry and want to eat more. On the other hand,

Figure A2-1

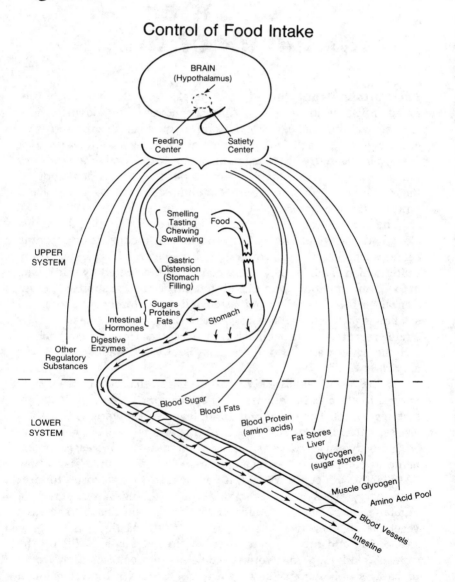

Control of Food Intake

even though lettuce has a fairly good blend of carbohydrates, fats and proteins, you would not be able to eat the 20 pounds necessary to meet your energy needs. Even though you would get enough chewing, tasting, swallowing and gastric distention to be totally satisfied, you would probably still receive strong messages to eat because the caloric content would be so low.

Ingesting 1000 calories in the form of straight carbohydrates would cause a similar problem, although the need for tasting, chewing, swallowing, and stomach distention would all be met. The lack of fats and proteins would cause a continued stimulation of the feeding center. As you can see, poorly balanced diets may provide enough calories, but still leave you hungry. An example of how powerful these drives can be is seen in patients suffering with bulimia who try to control weight by self-induced vomiting. By eating, they obtain the satisfaction that comes from chewing, tasting, swallowing and stomach distention. Because they induce vomiting, foods do not reach the intestines or the bloodstream and the feeding centers are strongly stimulated. Young girls have been know to eat $60 to $70 worth of food a day to satisfy their needs. One young bulimic lady who moved in with a family of six more than doubled the family food bill. At night she would get up to satisfy the strong urges she felt and would ingest a whole cake, several quarts of ice cream, huge volumes of leftover food and then would force herself to vomit. This particular method of weight control may cause severe electrolyte disturbances as well as a number of psychiatric problems. Although some people lose a little weight initially, bulimia is ineffective in the long run, and may actually induce severe obesity.

Several novel ideas have been developed in an attempt to overcome the body's controls and allow easy weight loss. One of these methods involves adding undigestible fiber to bread and other foods. Although a modest short-term reduction in calorie intake occurs, the sensing devices quickly detect that the food has fewer calories, and the hunger drive increases to protect the fat and prevent further weight loss.

Another attempt to fool the system involves using starch blockers. These products inhibit amylase, a digestive enzyme responsible for breaking down starches (long-chain sugars) into simple sugars so they can be digested. Since the amylase can't perform its usual function, the starches pass through the digestive system intact. The food intake regulators are quickly aware that these nutrients are not being absorbed, and the hunger drive increases to encourage more eating. The WRM can begin to conserve energy so that the body can still maintain weight at the lower nutrient intake. Although there may be a small amount of short-term weight loss, there is little evidence that starch blockers have any long-term effects.

The major concern with starch blockers is that the best possible fuel source (starch) is blocked, leaving most of the calories to be provided by sugars, fats and proteins. Most people already eat too many sugars, fats and proteins so starch blockers may decrease the nourishment available in the diet.

Another new product called polydextrose is a sugar substitute that has the texture and cooking properties of sugar, but is poorly absorbed, so that only one-fourth the calories of sugar are utilized. Here again there may be a small, short-term weight loss, but the body will soon sense the reduction and begin to conserve energy to balance the need.

None of these products will, by themselves, provide any significant long-term help for the overweight. The body has too many built-in protective mechanisms to be overcome by such simplistic approaches. Save your money until someone develops a product that can lower the setpoint.

As you have seen, the regulation of food intake is very complex and depends on many different factors. The weight-regulating mechanism can also sense short, mid-range, and long-term needs and adjusts the appetite to meet these needs. For instance, all of us have short-term needs in terms of dietary intake, but these needs must be modified to meet the mid- and long-range requirements as well. This section discusses the relationships between the various requirements and tells how the food intake regulator works to accomplish its task.

Short-term Control.

The short-term needs depend on 1) the composition or type of food eaten; 2) the efficiency of the body in absorbing that food; and, 3) the effect of insulin on the body.

1. Composition or Type of Food You Eat

The types of food eaten have a marked effect on the immediate satiety and how long that satiety will last. If all of the food in a meal was carbohydrate, it will quickly empty from the stomach and the control center will perceive a lack of fats and protein and request more food. Satiety will probably not occur and the sense of hunger will progressively increase. This will lead to a tendency to snack and will encourage you to eat the next meal sooner than usual.

If too little carbohydrate is consumed, the sugar needs of the body are not adequately met and you may be hungry again very soon. However, a very low carbohydrate diet sometimes suppresses hunger artificially because of the production of ketones. This type of dieting produces marked loss of water and has many other problems which will be discussed later.

If excess fats are eaten, the meal becomes calorically dense and too many calories will be consumed before the satiety needs are met. But fats do stimulate the release of cholecystokinin, an enzyme which delays the emptying of the stomach. Proteins are not used to a great extent for energy.

The form of the food eaten has a great effect on the appetite. For instance, sugar is called a disaccharide and has only two simple sugar molecules linked together. It can be broken quickly into single sugars or monosacharides by the action of the enzymes found in the saliva. Because it is broken down and dispersed quickly it can also be absorbed and enter the bloodstream quickly. Vegetables, cereals, and other "complex" carbohydrate foods are also composed of sugars, but these sugars are linked together like the links of a chain and may be several thousand sugar molecules long. These chains of sugars are mixed together with some undigestible fiber. Even though complex carbohydrates are chewed, the particles are much larger than the simple molecules found in refined sugar and it takes longer for the body to break them down into small enough pieces to be absorbed. This produces a steady, slow breakdown of sugar which is then gradually absorbed into the bloodstream instead of being absorbed within minutes as is refined sugar. Starches and compound sugars found in natural form may take three or four or more hours to be absorbed. The intestines can then act as a secondary storage unit for carbohydrates, and the release of sugar into the bloodstream is slowed dramatically as compared to simple sugar ingestion.

Fats are stored by plants and animals inside fat cells, as part of cell walls, or in other parts of the organism structure. Refined fats, such as vegetable oils, are squeezed out of the vegetable and are in a more or less purified form, which the body can quickly absorb.

Natural plant fats or animal fats require a lot of chewing and they enter the stomach in larger pieces, which slows the absorption process. Again, the intestines act as a storage unit releasing small amounts of fat into the bloodstream over a longer period of time. Therefore, purified or refined fats do not produce satiety for as long as fats contained in a more complex form.

Protein from most animal and plant sources is usually found in a complex form and is slow to be digested. Milk and milk products are exceptions and seem to be broken down more rapidly. Predigested protein liquids and powders are also more purified and can be absorbed more quickly. Processed powdered eggs, processed soybean flour and various kinds of milk powder may also be absorbed more quickly than complex proteins and they also have the potential to cause excess insulin production.

2. Efficiency of Absorption

There is some evidence that the surface area of the gut can be increased by food denial to increase the efficiency of absorption. This increased absorptive area comes about as a result of an increase in the size of the folds and finger-like projections of the intestinal lining. When food is absorbed quickly, the satiety period following a meal is shortened. The rapidly absorbed food can also be processed quickly, leading to hunger in a short time. Rapidly absorbed sugars may also lead to a sudden elevation in the blood sugar, which can stimulate increased insulin production. Rats eating only one meal a day have a markedly increased rate of food digestion and absorption. Many obese people also seem to digest food more quickly, perhaps because of dietary efforts and periods of food denial.

3. The Insulin Mechanism

Because of the importance of the insulin mechanism to weight control, it will be discussed in some detail at this point.

Insulin by itself will produce obesity with no extra eating required. As an example, if two groups of rats are exercised and fed the same, they would be expected to weigh the same. If one group is injected with insulin, that group becomes very fat. Although no extra food is needed for obesity to occur, extra insulin usually stimulates increased appetite as well.

Besides playing an important role in influencing the short-term food needs of the body, insulin also contributes to obesity in many other ways. Following is a detailed description of the role of insulin.

Insulin in Obesity

Insulin is an essential hormone that allows the cells of the body to take in and burn sugar from the bloodstream. When insufficient insulin is present, sugar can't enter the cells and blood glucose levels increase. This condition is called diabetes mellitis, or more commonly, diabetes. This type of diabetes is often referred to as Type I diabetes or insulin-dependent diabetes since extra insulin needs to be injected into the body so that the sugars can be used. In another form of diabetes, called adult maturity onset diabetes, non-insulin dependent diabetes, or Type II diabetes, there is enough insulin present, but for some reason the cells are resistant to the insulin and it is not effective in getting sugar into the cell.

Most obese people have some insulin resistance and are either diabetic or have a tendency toward diabetes. Because of this resistance, extra insulin is often produced. This excess insulin seems to cause many of the problems relative to obesity.

In the presence of excess insulin, a disproportionate share of the sugar in the bloodstream is converted to fat and deposited in the fat stores. Excess insulin also seems to inhibit or slow the breakdown of fats for the energy needs of the body. This combination leads to more reliance on sugar as the major fuel source, a more rapid use of the ingested sugars, the need for more frequent eating, the eating of larger volumes of food, and a preference for sugars in the diet. It also leads to an increase in fat stores and the protection of those fat stores.

There is good evidence that the obese and thin are quite different in the way they handle sugar. When the two groups eat sugar labeled with a radioactive substance, the thin quickly use the sugar for fuel. In obese people, however, most of the radioactive carbon stays within the body, presumably converted by the action of insulin into fat and stored within the body.

Figure A2.2 shows a glucose tolerance test comparing a typical obese person who has some degree of insulin resistance and a normal person. Because of the insulin resistance in the obese, the sugars are not taken up as quickly by the cells so the blood sugar levels rise rapidly to an abnormally high level. This rapid rise is a strong

Figure A2-2

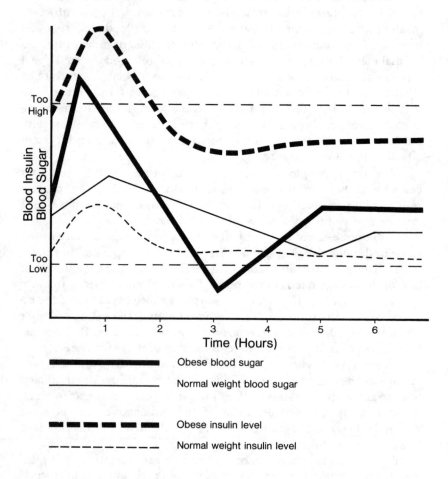

Effect of Obesity on Blood Sugar and Insulin

stimulus for insulin production, which then causes the blood sugar to fall much too rapidly and to unacceptably low levels. The body counters this fall in blood sugar by releasing a number of different hormones to restore proper sugar levels, but in the process the body's sugar stores are depleted. The obese person also has a limited ability to use fats for fuel. This is due in part to the role of high insulin levels in inhibiting fat breakdown from the fat stores, and a relative decrease in fat-metabolizing enzymes in the muscles compared to thin people. Since the sugar stores of the obese person are smaller and since he can't derive enough energy for his needs from the fat stores, he often becomes very tired and hungry. Hunger and tiredness can also occur as a result of rapidly falling blood sugar, or excessively low blood sugar levels. At any of these times the obese person may feel like he is out of fuel, that he desperately needs something to eat and is attracted to foods high in sugar or white flour. The feeling may not be so much hunger as it is a compensation to keep from getting weak, tired, shaky or for controlling other symptoms.

If the obese person eats in response to these hunger drives, he eats more calories than the body needs and fat gain can occur. The increased intake of sugar also tends to increase the setpoint.

If the obese person does not eat in response to these drives his body can't produce enough energy and he may feel very tired or weak. If he insists on being active, the protein from muscle tissue may be broken down to provide the extra energy needs. If this occurs very often or over a long period of time, a significant amount of muscle can be lost. Since metabolic rate is related to muscle mass, a loss of muscle tissue will decrease the metabolic rate and fewer calories will be burned than before. If this process continues, muscle mass is gradually lost and is replaced by fat so that the weight can remain the same. Losing muscle also seems to produce a decrease in endurance and strength.

Figure A2.3 shows in more detail the insulin effects seen in obesity. Note that the sugar is absorbed from the intestines more quickly in the obese person than in the normal weight person. This also contributes to the rapid rise in blood sugar level that stimulates excess insulin production. The arrows from the intestines depict that a disproportionate share of sugar is converted to fat in the obese person and stored in the fat stores. Although some sugar is diverted to sugar stores, these stores are rather limited compared to the normal

Figure A2-3
Insulin Effect in Obesity

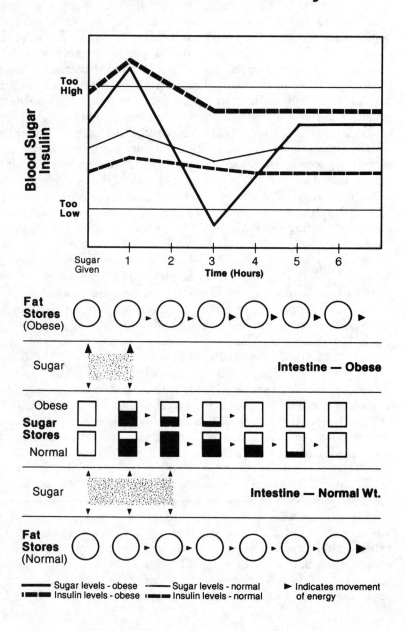

weight person. The normal weight person seems to derive about half of his energy from sugar and half from fat (depicted by the arrows leading away from sugar and fat stores). Because of insulin resistance and diminished fat-burning enzymes, the obese person seems to derive a disproportionate share of energy from the sugar stores (note the relative size of the arrows leading from fat and sugar stores). With reduced sugar stores to begin with and excess reliance on these stores for energy, with sugar in the intestines quickly absorbed, and with high levels of insulin driving sugar from the bloodstream, the obese person soon depletes the sugar stores. Although the normal weight person can merely increase the use of fat for energy when sugar stores are depleted, the obese person has a limited ability to do this. The result is hunger (especially a specific hunger for sugar), tiredness, and weakness. The obese person will then usually move slowly and conserve energy. The body may derive the needed energy from breaking down muscle stores.

The ability of the obese to conserve the fat and utilize muscle is a very effective defense against starvation and allows the use of muscle for some of the energy needs. It may also account for the tendency of overweight people to lose large amounts of weight during the early stages of a diet, then little or none during later stages. When muscle is used for energy instead of fat, weight can be lost about ten times as fast. A pound of protein has less than one-half the energy of one pound of fat, and muscle is one part protein mixed with four parts water. Each pound of muscle, then, has only one-tenth the energy of fat. This muscle loss is very counterproductive, since it leaves you with a more efficient body which has less energy, strength and endurance than before, often with the unsightly fat still in place.

There are other factors known to affect insulin, which in turn affects obesity. Because these factors are so important, they will be discussed briefly below:

- Intake of refined carbohydrates (e.g., sugars and white flour). Refined sugars are absorbed very quickly, causing a rapid increase in blood sugar which acts as a very strong stimulus for high levels of insulin production.
- Refined protein (pre-digested protein liquid or powder, processed powdered eggs, etc.). With refined protein, amino acid levels rise quickly in the blood and can act as strong insulin stimulators.

- Caffeine intake. Caffeine is a strong insulin stimulator. This may be due to a direct insulin stimulation, or as a result of the high levels of sugars released into the blood when caffeine is ingested.
- Eating irregular meals. Long periods with no eating seem to interfere with glucose metabolism by increasing insulin resistance. An interesting study done in England a few years ago divided a large group of men into those eating one meal a day, those eating two, and those eating three or more meals per day. The study showed that those eating one meal a day had more insulin resistance than those eating several meals a day. Incidentally, those eating one meal a day were also heavier, and had higher cholesterol levels as well.
- Low carbohydrate intake. For some reason low carbohydrate intake interferes with glucose metabolism by increasing insulin resistance.
- Lack of exercise. Exercise exerts a direct suppressant effect on insulin levels and reduces insulin resistance.
- Fat cell size. Large fat cells seen in the obese person somehow produce insulin resistance. As the fat cell size is reduced with an effective weight-management program, insulin resistance decreases.
- Trace metal deficiencies. Deficiencies in chromium, potassium, magnesium, and zinc may cause insulin resistance or high insulin levels. The reason for this is not entirely clear, but the evidence is fairly strong that it does happen.
- Other hormones. A number of hormones including adrenal control hormones (cortisone), estrogen, and progesterone seem to cause some insulin resistance. Cortisone, in particular, often brings on diabetes in those with borderline diabetes, and this mechanism may account for the weight gain so often seen with cortisone use.
- Dietary fats. It has been theorized that fats in the diet have a profound influence on insulin resistance. Evidence for this comes mainly from experimental diets involving very low fat levels. These high fiber, low fat diets have been shown to greatly decrease the diabetic's need for insulin. Some of the effect may come from the high fiber, high nutrient part of the diet, and some from the decrease in fats. Whatever the factor, fats do seem to have an effect on insulin resistance.

You can see from the above information that insulin is very important in obesity. It directs much of the sugar into fat production, it decreases the amount of sugar stores, and it decreases the ability of the body cells to use fat for fuel. The action of insulin stimulates other hormones which further break down sugar stores. All of these factors shorten the satiety period after a meal. Insulin also increases the drive for more sugar intake and this causes a generalized hunger as well as a specific hunger for sweets.

Mid-Range Controls

Mid-range controls seem to balance out our energy needs for one day or so. The function of the mid-range controls can perhaps best be seen in those eating only one meal per day. The typical dieter may go all day eating little or no food and then eat too fast and too much with the evening meal and feel the need to snack later in the evening. This occurs because the mid-range regulators sense the need for the entire day's energy requirements to be supplied only in the evening. This often causes more eating than the stomach can comfortably hold and stimulates extra snacking after the meal to ensure satisfactory intake. Even though he may still be so full an hour or two after the meal that he feels uncomfortable, the one-meal-a-day eater will still feel the need to snack frequently afterward to compensate for having missed food all day. The mid-range needs will tell him that he has a need for more food which he will attempt to take in before the day is over. This response is typical for normal weight people who miss meals as well as for overweight people.

Long-Range Controls

The control of food intake over the long-range from several days to several months depends on certain measured information from the body, such as the size of the fat cells, the amount of fat storage, protein storage, and the total body weight. This information is fed back to the long-range part of the feeding control mechanism. An example of this can occur with the force-feeding studies previously mentioned. When the studies are over, the weight is higher than the weight chosen by the weight-regulating mechanism, and with no attempt to diet, the person will automatically decrease his food intake and soon lose the excess weight. If the long-range control sensors detect a higher than normal weight or an increase in fat storage, the message is sent to the food intake centers to decrease the stimulation to the feeding center or to increase the stimulation of the satiety center or both. If the long-range control were the only control, no eating would occur until the body weight and fat storage returned to the present levels. Because of the short-term needs, some eating will still occur. The person may eat a little less each meal and may eat a little less often until the weight returns to former levels.

If a person tries to lose weight below the weight-regulating mechanism setpoint, the body will quickly detect that the weight is dropping, that the fat cell size is decreasing and that there is a total reduction in the fat stores. This center then produces a stimulation in the feeding mechanism and a decrease in the stimulation of the satiety centers or both. The subject then experiences increased hunger or even a rather constant desire to eat, until the deficit is made up. In this case, the short-term and long-term needs act together to induce more frequent and larger meals. These hunger drives may manifest themselves by the person opening the refrigerator door six times a night, thinking more about food and being generally obsessed with eating.

Appendix Three
How the Body Wastes and Conserves Energy

For many years, scientific thinking related to obesity has centered around one of the Laws of Thermodynamics. This law simply states that energy input equals energy output. It has been theorized that if you eat less food than your body needs, you will burn your fat stores for fuel and lose weight. This has led us to blame overeating as the major cause of obesity and has stimulated the development of hundreds of diets and other techniques to control how much we eat.

The trouble with this approach is that it doesn't explain what is actually observed in relation to the problem. For instance, we all have a relative or friend who "eats like a horse" but doesn't gain an ounce. On the other extreme, we all know people who claim to eat only a few calories but still remain extremely fat. Force feeding studies have substantiated these observations. Large increases in food intake will usually cause some increase in body weight, but only to a point. After about a 14 percent weight gain, most people level off, even if they continue eating excessive amounts of food. Some people fail to gain weight even though they eat enough extra food to theoretically gain several pounds a week.

It is difficult to explain why some people fail to gain weight and others gain only a moderate amount and level off, unless you hypothesize some kind of energy- wasting system. This seems to be exactly what happens. The WRM obviously exerts a powerful influence on the body to waste the energy supplied by excessive food as the weight climbs above the setpoint. After a prolonged period of excessive food intake, the body may actually improve its ability to waste energy.

An exact reversal of this process occurs in people who stay fat on small quantities of food. There are documented studies of overweight adults who maintain their weight on fewer than 1000 calories per day. These adults are obviously able to conserve energy so efficiently that fat cells are not depleted by restricted intakes of food. Again, the ability to conserve energy is probably also developed with constant dieting or true starvation. In fact, the body probably can't tell the difference between the two.

This mechanism makes good sense in terms of adaptive response to protect life. In periods of hard times when little food is available, the ability to conserve energy may make the difference between life and death.

Energy Conservation and Wasting.

The question, then, is "What is the mechanism the body uses to waste or conserve energy?" There are several known factors that can explain how energy conservation and wasting occur. We think that it is important that you understand how this is accomplished, so we will discuss each of these factors in some detail in the following section:

Basal Metabolic Rate. The most well-known factor that can be used to conserve or waste energy is a change in the basal metabolic rate (BMR) of the body. The BMR reflects the energy required to support the basic resting functions of life (heart rate, breathing, brain and neural activity, organ function, etc.).

Scientists have long known that food affects the metabolic rate. If you eat just prior to checking the rate, it will be higher than if you are fasting. On the other hand, restricted food intake for a period of time will decrease the metabolic rate dramatically. This effect of food is called (in rather scientific terms) "The Specific Dynamic Action of Food."

Activity also affects BMR. Athletes and those who perform heavy manual labor have extremely high metabolic rates. Not only do they use more energy during their activity period, but their resting metabolism is higher as well.

Time-motion studies show that overweight people use even less energy doing simple tasks like making a bed; the average thin woman moves around the bed several times, while the overweight woman tends to accomplish more from the same position. It is as if the obese person is directed by the control centers to conserve energy in every way possible, to move more slowly, to work more efficiently, and to rest more often.

Even at rest the average obese person conserves energy. Grossly obese people often sit for prolonged periods, hardly moving a muscle. In contrast, thin people often shift around in their chair, cross and uncross the legs and arms, tap the feet and fingers, and get up and walk around. It is as if these people were driven to waste energy through some type of unproductive movement.

It is probably not the degree of fatness that affects the amount of movement. It is probably the body's perceived need to either waste or conserve energy. Since obese people usually are trying to control their weight and are often dieting in an attempt to do so, their bodies are often programmed to an energy conservation mode. Those people who are living at a weight level lower than that set by the WRM may also exhibit energy conservation traits.

Brown Fat. One of the most exciting finds in modern obesity research was the presence of brown fat stores in the human body. Brown fat is unlike regular or white fat in that rather than being primarily a storage depot for excess energy, it has a high metabolic activity potential. In fact, the brownish color probably comes from blood flow and chemicals within the cell that aid metabolic activity.

Brown fat has been studied in animals for some time. Found mostly in hibernators, it is probably activated to help restore them to normal temperature after the long hibernation period and as a "metabolic warming blanket" against cooling of the body in a cold environment. This tissue in animals is full of blood vessels and has such a high metabolic rate that in rats it can account for a five-fold increase in resting heat production. It can also hypertrophy and become more effective if needed.

Although not as much is known about the role of brown fat in humans, there is evidence that the obese have less total brown fat storage and that it is much less active. Obviously, at least some excess energy could be "burned" in this "heating blanket" of metabolically active tissue and this energy would then be released as heat rather than stored as fat.

Apparently, this is one of the reasons that thin people who eat a lot stay thin. In fact, these people may actually increase their brown fat stores so that they can waste more and more energy. On the other hand, people who have a poor supply of or inactive brown fat may store fat effectively because there is no brown fat to waste it.

Sodium-Potassium Pump Activity. Another way the body can waste energy is through the use of a system called the sodium-potassium pump. This pump is found in each of the trillions of cells in the body and is used to maintain a slight electrical charge at the cell membrane so that the cell can be told what to do. An enzyme called sodium-potassium ATP-ase is required for the release of energy for the pump and the level of this enzyme is related to the amount of pump activity.

It has been shown experimentally that obese people have a lower level of this enzyme than normal and are therefore unable to waste as much energy as normal weight people.

Remember, if energy isn't used through physical activity, or basal metabolic activity, it must be stored as fat. Unless, of course, you have some "futile" cycles such as brown fat or the sodium-potassium pump that can "use up" excess fat and release it as heat. A decreased sodium-potassium pump activity may also affect the potassium level in the cells and cause some of the insulin resistance seen in the obese.

Appendix Four
Factors Contributing to Obesity

In this appendix, we will discuss the various factors which contribute to obesity. We will show how these factors work by changing the setpoint to a higher level, or by overpowering the weight-regulating mechanism, causing more food intake than the body can waste, leaving no alternative but to store the extra energy as fat. We will discuss other factors in the model of obesity in Appendix 12 that may not directly affect the weight-regulating mechanism, but do contribute to the problem.

This material is presented as a background to treatment principles discussed in the main text of the book. By having a correct understanding of the obesity process, you will be much more likely to make intelligent choices, follow proper management principles, and ultimately succeed in your weight control efforts. With this in mind, we classify obesity-inducing factors into those you cannot change, those you can change to a limited extent, and those over which you have complete control.

Factors Beyond Control

Genetics. It is obvious that you cannot change your genetic makeup. Research has shown that inheritance has a powerful influence over both our body build and our tendency toward obesity. Studies have shown that if both of your parents are obese, there is an 80 percent chance of you becoming obese. Studies of twins separated at birth show that genetic makeup is more important than environment in producing obesity.

Having a genetic tendency toward obesity does not necessarily doom you to a life of obesity. Our genes work by controlling the various hormones, enzymes, and metabolic processes in the body. As we will show, many of these processes can be altered. The action of your genes can then be somewhat modified.

Events that Have Already Taken Place

You cannot exert any influence over events that have already occurred, i.e., episodes of dieting, taking certain drugs and hormones, inactivity, pregnancy, and old stresses.

Controlling obesity may not be as easy as merely reversing some past behavior. If you have led a very stressful life, learning to have a stress-free life may improve the situation, but may not reverse the obesity process.

Fat Cell Number. We have mentioned that obesity can occur as a result of increased fat cell size, increased fat cell numbers or both. If some factor in your life has produced an increased number of fat cells, a reversal of that factor will not decrease the number of fat cells, and fat loss will be more difficult. For instance, a long distance runner can get his body fat content down to 3 to 5 percent of his body weight. Since most runners usually have a normal number of fat cells, each cell must be quite small for such a decrease in total body fat to occur. A man with three times as many fat cells as the distance runner may be 15 percent fat even if the fat cells were as small as the distance runner's. People who have become grossly obese may have so many excess fat cells that becoming lean and staying lean may be much more difficult.

Factors That Can be Partially Controlled

Hormones. There are many hormonal differences between the obese and those of normal weight. Most of these hormones exert at least part of their effect by either increasing insulin resistance, or increasing insulin production. Either way, these changes tend to enhance energy conservation, which in turn produces the other problems related to excessive insulin levels. The most involved include adrenal steroids (mainly cortisol), growth hormones, low thyroid levels, aldosterone, and progestational agents.

The adrenal cortical hormones (cortisol and cortisone) have effects on obesity other than increasing insulin resistance. They seem to directly change the setpoint to a higher level. An increased production of adrenal corticosteroid (cortisol and cortisone) causes Cushing's Syndrome, which is almost always associated with obesity. Even giving cortisone to a patient for the treatment of a medical problem will usually cause weight gain. Corticosteroids also cause a breakdown of muscle tissue. This makes the body conserve energy more effectively.

The hormone aldosterone increases insulin resistance and plays a role in fluid retention. It tends to encourage potassium excretion (which increases insulin resistance) and helps retain sodium. This may be the method by which aldosterone leads to fluid retention and high blood pressure. Both these problems are found with greater frequency in the obese population. The retention of fluid also accounts for some of the weight seen in obese people. Rapid weight losses at the beginning of most dieting efforts may be predominantly loss of this extra fluid and not fat.

Fluid retention is often treated with a diuretic, or "water pill." Most of these products cause potassium loss, which actually makes the obesity problem worse by creating more insulin resistance. There are a number of other hormones found in abnormal levels in the obese population. The exact mechanism by which these hormones contribute to obesity is uncertain. Research will probably identify these hormonal problems in the future so we can control them. Many hormones in the body are interrelated, and changes in one hormone seem to affect the levels of other hormones. Some of these hormonal imbalances will revert to normal when insulin is controlled and weight is reduced. Others remain abnormal, and may be a prime factor in the extremely common tendency for weight to be regained after dieting.

Of all the hormones in the body, the thyroid hormone has been most studied with relation to the problem of obesity. However, its role is still unclear. The results of early studies have indicated that using thyroid hormone may be an effective weight-loss technique. However, more recent research has shown that most of the extra weight loss is from protein tissue, and not fat. The protein loss is mainly from the muscle tissue and results in decreased strength, endurance, and energy levels, and leaves the body more energy efficient. Thyroid hormone also has its dangers, and its use for treating obesity in people with normal thyroid function has been specifically condemned by the F.D.A. Even in patients with low thyroid function, giving thyroid hormone does not automatically correct the weight problem. In our experience, using thyroid in these cases provides very little help with weight, even though people feel better when thyroid levels are regulated properly.

A newly discovered hormone, prostaglandin E1, about which little is known, may play a significant role in the control of fat. Prostaglandin E1 is thought to be related to brown fat and sodium-potassium pump activity. Low levels of this hormone may be related to energy conservation.

Prostaglandin E1 is formed from gamma linoleic which is made from an essential fatty acid. The step from linoleic acid to gamma linoleic acid may be blocked by high levels of saturated fats or certain forms of polyunsaturated fats. The average American diet, which is high in fat, may reduce prostaglandin E1 and make it more difficult to lose weight. One of the new treatment possibilities is taking gamma linoleic acid to increase the production of prostaglandin E1. A better way would be to reduce the fats that block the prostaglandin production. However, this whole area requires much more research before we really understand the role of the prostaglandins.

Dieting and Starvation The practice of dieting (restricting the number of calories eaten) and starvation (going without food for a period of time) to control weight may be a major factor in obesity, since an inadequate intake of food triggers the body's starvation defenses. As a result, the setpoint goes up, you get hungrier, your body begins to conserve energy, and certain biochemical changes occur that help you store fat effectively. One of the major biochemical changes relates to the role of an enzyme called lipoprotein lipase (LPL). This enzyme plays a major role in the development and maintenance of obesity because it helps fat cells pick up and store fat. A recent study showed the effect of dieting on LPL. The LPL levels were dramatically higher in subjects who had lost weight by dieting. When these subjects returned to their original weight, the LPL levels also returned to normal. It was almost as if the body was increasing LPL in a counter-regulatory attempt to return the reduced fat mass back to its original obese state.

In rats, the tendency to respond to decreased food intake is so strong that it occurs even at the expense of other body tissue. In another study, one group of genetically obese rats was allowed to eat freely and the second group had a restricted food intake. Although the first group became heavier, the second group actually had a higher percent body fat. These deprived rats had only 1/2 the muscle tissue of the fed rats, and even the brain and kidneys weighed less. The tendency to preserve fat stores at the expense of lean tissue during dieting is also observed in people. Obviously, it would be better to avoid these responses if possible.

Drugs. Certain drugs have been reported in the medical literature to be associated with weight gain. Anti-inflammatory and antidepressant drugs are particularly prone to cause fat gain, presumably by changing the setpoint to a higher level. In some cases, with the approval of your doctor, the drugs can be stopped or changed. In other cases, it may be best to continue the drugs. Following the proper exercise and management principles may partly counteract the effect of these drugs.

Stress. Stress contributes to obesity in several ways. It seems to directly change the setpoint. An interesting experiment with rats showed that obesity results from the stress induced by frequent painful tail pinching. Stress often seems to be associated with the beginning or worsening of human obesity as well. The stress hormones also produce insulin resistance, which in turn, leads to excess insulin production, fat deposits, and inhibition of fat breakdown.

Many people eat excessively in response to stress since food can have a relaxing effect. The release of some stress hormones often occurs when the body is in need of sugars. You can develop a conditioned response so that whenever stress hormone levels become high, you feel the need to eat.

None of us can control our stress completely, but we can reduce stress to some extent. Much attention has recently been focused on stress management techniques to promote better health.

Environment. Many of the factors that lead to obesity result from our association with other people within our environment. For instance, you often learn certain food preference patterns, favoring highly seasoned or sweet foods, or develop a taste and habit for dessert from the types of food you ate as a child. You even learn to eat fast or slow or to eat early or late because of these influences. Our interest and participation in active sports or activities is also to some extent learned as is the way we handle stress and stress-producing situations.

Although the environment cannot be completely controlled, we can learn new ways of responding. By identifying the problem areas, and attempting to change only those aspects of your life that are producing problems, you should be much more successful than if you blindly try to change a whole group of behaviors, many of which have no bearing at all on your particular eating or weight problem.

Minerals. A decrease in the level of certain minerals can have an effect on fat storage. For instance, the mineral zinc is found in some of the enzymes involved in sugar metabolism. These enzymes are necessary for the metabolic processing of sugars in order to release energy for the body's needs. It has recently been suggested that in a deficiency of zinc, sugars tend to be only partly metabolized. The partly metabolized sugar is channeled into the fat production cycle where it eventually becomes part of the fat stores of the body. This is a beautiful adaptive mechanism. The body, when faced with starvation and lack of dietary zinc, will soon stop burning off the sugars and direct them to fat stores. This ability confers survival value during famine conditions. Unfortunately, it also conserves energy during dietary periods with poor nutritional intake. This may be one more reason why some obese people have trouble providing enough energy for themselves, and are usually tired.

A recent study in a pediatrics weight loss group showed that a number of children with low zinc levels did not lose weight at the expected rate. When treated with adequate zinc supplements, weight loss then proceeded at the normal rate.

A decrease in the body's other minerals levels (potassium, chromium, magnesium, etc.) can also cause problems. Many of these minerals increase cellular resistance to the action of insulin.

This insulin resistance seen with low mineral levels is a very effective adaptation to starvation. When inadequate minerals are available, the body naturally turns to energy conservation to protect the organism. This mechanism has probably helped many of our ancestors survive famines. Unfortunately, eating foods of poor nutritional quality during a restrictive diet also seems to trigger this mechanism.

Factors that can be Effectively Controlled

Inactivity. One of the easiest and most effective changes we can make in our lives, and one over which we have complete control, is becoming active. The major reason for increasing activity is that it can and does move the setpoint to a lower level. A good example of this effect is seen in seasonal workers. During the seven or eight months of the year that they engage in hard physical labor, they stabilize at a lean low-fat body build. However, during the off-season, they often increase and stabilize at a higher weight. This may happen year after year. If these men change to a more regular but inactive job, they often become and remain obese.

In the same way, a wild rat has low body fat content, but when put in a laboratory cage will become mildly obese, perhaps comparable to a person who is 20 to 30 pounds overweight. This mild obesity is normal for an inactive rat and he will become lean again if he is exercised. Surprisingly, the food intake of the rat actually decreases when he is exercised even though his energy requirements increase. This finding would suggest that the weight loss is not just due to extra calories lost through exercise, but rather that the setpoint is lowered and the body adjusts the appetite to the new setting. People who exercise notice much the same response. Even though they make no attempt whatever to adjust their food intake, they will usually eat less and their weight will drop to a lower level and then stabilize itself. When the weight stablizes, the food intake may increase again to prevent further weight loss.

The level of the setpoint seems to depend to a large extent on the amount of exercise done. People who exercise moderately lower their body fat to a reasonable level and then lose no further. People who exercise more strenuously lose considerably more fat. Perhaps the best example is the long-distance runner. He makes no attempt to juggle his intake, but because of the massive amount of exercise, the weight-regulating mechanism seems satisfied to maintain a body fat percentage of only 3 to 4 percent. People who control their weight through exercise alone often notice an almost immediate gain if they are forced to quit exercising because of illness or injury. The setpoint can be adjusted to varying levels depending on the activity level.

Another problem with inactivity relates to a loss of muscle tissue. This is a natural body reaction that allows a person to decrease the size of a nonfunctioning limb so it can be moved more easily. The most graphic example of this is the size decrease seen in an arm or leg when it has been in a cast. This same effect is seen in astronauts after even short space flights. They begin to lose protein and calcium and decrease their muscle mass because of the decreased gravitational pull.

Of course, a decreased muscle mass yields a decreased basal metabolic rate and decreases the ability of the body to burn fat at rest or during work.

Inactivity is a problem of modern life. Children now watch TV instead of participating in games and activities. Adults have a similar problem. Machines do much of the work that was formerly done by hand. A higher percentage of jobs now are inactive "desk jobs." In the home, labor-saving devices promote inactivity. Even jobs traditionally requiring hard physical labor are now much less physically demanding because of machines.

Increased Fat Intake. One of the biggest problems contributing to obesity is the amount of fat in the diet. The average North American consumes about 40 to 50 percent of his calories in the form of fat, and there is evidence that excessive fat intake affects the setpoint. In experimental rats, a modest increase in fat intake will produce obesity Even rats that have had the feeding center surgically destroyed will gain weight with increased dietary fats. It is as if the body recognizes that fat has a high caloric density and increases the setpoint to help put it into storage for rainy days ahead. This process is like buying extra items for storage while they are on sale.

Ingested fats can be efficiently converted into stored fat. This process requires fewer steps and less energy than converting dietary sugar and protein into fat. A study comparing the effects of a high-carbohydrate diet to one high in fat showed that the high-fat group converted about twice as many of the ingested calories into body fat.

Another possible explanation for the influence of dietary fats in producing obesity involves its influence on taste. High fat foods taste good, and the texture is pleasurable. (Cheese-cake fans will know what we mean.) Both rats and people will eat high fat foods for taste and pleasure even when they are not hungry. Of course, these extra calories are then easily stored in the fat cells.

Fats also have a much higher caloric density than other foods. That is, they contain more than twice as many calories per gram than do carbohydrates and proteins (fats - 9 KCal/gram; carbohydrates and proteins - 4 KCal/gram). They also contain much less water than carbohydrates and protein. For instance, fruits and vegetables (carbohydrates) are from 70 to 95 percent water, and most protein sources are probably 70 to 80 percent water. Fats, on the other hand, usually have from 0 to 15 percent water content. This means that the "bulk" of fatty food is much less than that of other foods. For example, one pound of vegetable oil contains the same number of calories as 77 pounds of lettuce (about 4,000 calories). This is also equal (in calories) to 37 pounds of beans or 15 pounds of potatoes. There is certainly a lot more chewing, tasting, swallowing, and stomach distention to satisfy your hunger needs when you eat bulkier foods than when you consume fat. Diets high in fat almost always lead to too many calories.

Fats are also usually liquid or at least rather soft. They can be eaten with very little chewing and can be swallowed rather easily with little need for dilution or lubrication from salivary secretions. If you were to reduce the fat percentage of ingested food from 40 to 20 percent, and replace the fat with foods having a lower caloric density, you would be able to greatly increase the volume of food intake without adding any calories, or eat the same volume with a decrease in total calories.

Fats are also low in vitamins and minerals relative to the total number of calories they contain. Eating high fat meals may elevate the setpoint to ensure sufficient intake of food in order to provide adequate nutrients.

In rats, a high fat diet will dramatically decrease spontaneous activity. The same phenomenon occurs in people. We have all experienced the feeling of lethargy and desire for inactivity after a high fat meal. This decreased activity may play a profound role in producing and maintaining the obese state.

Refined Carbohydrates. The ingestion of refined carbohydrates (sugar, white flour, etc.) can contribute to obesity by raising the set-point to a higher level. The body must recognize "sweetness" as an opportunity to produce extra fat in case of future "hard times." Artificial sweeteners are probably not much better. Rats given artificial sweeteners in their water actually increased their food intake and gained weight. In our experience, those drinking diet pop seem to have a problem losing weight despite a rather restrictive caloric intake. This observation needs further study, but may implicate sweeteners in setpoint changes.

Refined carbohydrates also stimulate insulin production because they are absorbed so quickly. Insulin not only has a direct effect on the setpoint, it also increases hunger. Of course, when carbohydrates are refined, their caloric density is increased. Whereas most complex carbohydrates are from 80 to 95 percent water, refined sugar is less than 1 percent and white flour is only about 12 percent. When many calories are packed into a small volume, there is a tendency to consume too many calories, especially when they are prepared in a way that requires very little chewing. Sweets (refined carbohydrates) are also eaten for taste and pleasure. This usually results in overeating and eating without a hunger drive. You may also continue eating sweet things long after you feel satisfied, just because they taste good.

Both table sugar and white flour lose most of their nutrients when they are processed. Fortified flour has some of the vitamins replaced, but certainly not all of the nutrients that are removed in the milling process are restored. The ingestion of foods with empty calories may play a major role in producing obesity. The body seems to sense deficiencies in basic nutrients and overeating is the result.

Besides leading to extra eating, the ingestion of empty calories may actually lead to vitamin and mineral deficiencies. Deficiency of certain minerals leads to insulin resistance. This in turn causes excess insulin production with its inherent tendency to produce obesity. Zinc and other mineral deficiencies may also slow the breakdown of nutrients in the energy cycles, leading to conservation of energy and difficulty in losing weight.

Appendix Five
Exercises
That Can Be Used
for Weight Control

We would like to discuss several of the major activities that can be used for weight control, with specific suggestions and guidelines to help you use these activities more effectively.

Walking

Walking is the simplest and easiest of all the activities. It is a low-intensity activity and requires no special equipment or exercise area. Almost anyone can walk because the weight of the body is shared by the legs between steps. Therefore, walking causes few musculoskeletal problems. Research has shown that the cardiovascular endurance changes that occur in walkers are the same as occur in those who jog or ride bicycles. However, walkers must double the total duration to reap equal benefits.

There are no special rules for walking. You can walk in almost any weather, and you will surely enjoy the fresh air and scenery when the weather is good. Another advantage of walking is that it is easy to find someone to walk with you. Joggers must have comparable fitness levels to really enjoy running together; however, almost everyone walks at about the same speed.

We recommend comfortable shoes and loose-fitting clothes as the basic uniform. Many walkers end up buying a good pair of jogging shoes because they are so comfortable. However, they are not at all necessary.

Begin your program by walking about 20 minutes a day. Maintain this level for a week or two until you are sure that the muscles and joints are responding normally. Increase the time by five minutes a week or five minutes every two weeks (depending on your age and conditioning level) until you are walking an hour each day.

Jogging

Jogging is an excellent activity that can be done without expensive equipment or facilities. However, it will probably be too intense to be used effectively for weight control until you have lost a significant amount of weight and have devloped your fitness level through some lower intensity activity.

After you have been walking an hour a day for some time, you may want to begin jogging for short periods of time until you get breathless. At this point, slow to a walk until you recover. As you become more fit, the periods of jogging will increase and the periods of walking will decrease until you are jogging the entire time.

Just as there are no correct or incorrect ways to walk, there are no correct or incorrect ways to jog. You will surely develop your own jogging style. However, the following suggestions may be useful:

Stand up straight, keeping your back as straight as is naturally comfortable. Keep your head level. (Don't look at your feet.) Hold your arms slightly away from your body with the elbows bent about 90 degrees. The hands should be carried somewhere near the waist, and the arms can be straightened from time to time to help reduce tension in the shoulders. Keep the hands relaxed.

Run with a smooth, rolling motion, using moderate stride length. Try to land on the heel or entire bottom of your foot rather than on the ball or front part of the foot. The key is to reduce the impact as much as possible to avoid injury to the musculoskeletal system.

Keep your steps short by letting the foot strike the ground beneath the knee instead of reaching out in front of you. Remember, the slower the rate of running, the shorter the stride length should be.

Breathe through your mouth, and allow the rhythm of breathing to adjust naturally to your running rhythm.

If for some reason, known or unknown, you become unusually tired or uncomfortable while jogging, slow down to a walk, or stop. If you jog up a hill, slow down so that the heart rate is no greater going up than it was on the level. If necessary, walk for a while to keep the intensity comfortable for your fitness level.

What to Wear. The most important equipment for any runner is a pair of good quality, properly fitted running shoes. You will run hundreds of miles in the shoes you buy, so select them carefully. The sole should be flexible and the heel elevated and well-supported to prevent foot movement in the shoe while you run. Be sure that the toe box on the shoe is high enough to prevent rubbing on the tops of the toes. A low toe box will cause many problems, especially if you run down hills occasionally. The sole and heel material should be able to absorb most of the shock of the heel strike and should wear well. Luckily, several jogging magazines rate shoes annually for these and other factors. We recommend that you check the most current shoe ratings in *Runner's World* magazine. Most good sporting-goods stores or running-shoe stores will have a copy for your use. Any shoe that is in the top two categories or ratings and fits you will be a good investment.

Clothing should be comfortable and reasonably loose and should not restrict free movement of the arms or legs. Avoid tight-fitting clothing or clothing with tight elastic bands that restrict the return of blood from the extremities. Men need not wear athletic supporters; they sometimes irritate or chafe the skin. However, some support should be provided. Women should wear a running bra or a bra that provides adequate support.

In the summer, wear light clothes that will allow sweat to evaporate. You should never wear plastic or rubberized "sauna suits." These interfere with normal cooling and can cause body temperature to rise to dangerous levels.

In the winter, wear several layers of light clothing to increase the insulation. You should also wear cotton gloves and a warm hat that covers your ears. We often wear a towel or scarf around the neck to retain body heat. We also recommend a jogging suit with a zippered top rather than the pullover type. It is easy to adjust the heat by zipping up more or less as the weather changes or as you run into or with the wind.

If you must run along roads at dusk or at night, be sure to sew reflective tape to your suit.

Where to Jog. There is no restriction in terms of where to run, but it is a good idea for the beginner to run on grass if possible. This will allow the joints and muscles to toughen up with less strain. In fact, it is always best to choose the softest surface available to run on. Golf courses, jogging trails, parks, and similar places are excellent. However, some softer surfaces are irregular and could cause turned ankles or falls. If you do run on roads, always run facing traffic. If you are going to get hit, it is nice to know who hit you. Be sure to give the right of way to cars, bicycles, dogs, and pedestrians.

When to Jog. Almost any time of the day is acceptable for jogging - except an hour or so after meals and when the weather is extremely hot. We enjoy jogging just before lunch or before dinner in the evening. Many people love to get up early and jog before breakfast. Any schedule that allows you to be consistent will yield nice results.

Since jogging tends to tighten the muscles on the back side of the legs, we recommend that you do flexibility exercises regularly to maintain muscle length.

Swimming

Swimming is one of the most outstanding activities for developing cardiovascular fitness, but is only an average activity for losing weight. It involves all the major mucle groups of the body and is very rhythmic, and can be used by people unable to jog or walk because of a skeletal or structural problem. The buoyancy of the water reduces joint trauma to almost nothing. We have often used this activity for those with rheumatoid arthritis and other debilitating disease of the body structure.

The biggest drawback is that swimming requires a pool. If you do not have access to a pool or if you live where winter makes swimming impossible, you will have difficulty using this activity.

As with all activities, you need to start out slowly and increase the intensity as you become trained. If you are a swimmer, you should probably start by swimming lengths of the pool using a breaststroke or some other restful stroke and continue slowly for twenty minutes. If you are successful, you can slowly increase the intensity of some portions of the swim or change strokes from time to time, returning to the basic stroke if you get breathless. Work to complete the entire 20 minutes without stopping, even if you need to swim slowly on your back for part of the time. As you become more fit, you will probably swim some laps using the overhand crawl or another high-intensity stroke, alternating with easier strokes so that you can swim the whole time. You will soon swim more of the more intense strokes and less of the resting stroke as you progress in your efforts. You should check your heart rate from time to time to evaluate the intensity of the effort.

Nonswimmers can exercise effectively by walking back and forth in the four- to five-feet-deep area of the pool. To involve more muscle mass, you may wish to pull with the arms as you walk. As in other activities, start slowly so that you can continue for the entire duration,and increase the intensity for short periods as you become more fit. Check the heart rate from time to time to evaluate the intensity. Nonswimmers who exercise in the pool often begin swimming some laps and become good swimmers in time. All swimmers should have an alternate form of exercise because of the difficulty of always having a pool available.

Bicycling

Bicycling is also an excellent activity for fitness and weight control. The movement of the legs as they turn the pedals moves the blood effectively and efficiently back to the heart. Bicycling is enjoyable because you can cover a long distance in a fairly short time. This increases the fun because of the changes in scenery and the exhilaration associated with speed.

You can get an effective workout whether you use an expensive 10-speed or a cheap 3-speed bicycle. All that is required is that you keep the heart rate between 70 and 80 percent of your maximum.

You should begin by riding easily for about 20 minutes: ten minutes away from home and ten back. If you come to a hill too steep for you to ride up comfortably, get off and push your bike. After you have ridden for several weeks to toughen the upper legs, you can begin to check your pulse periodically. You should use the gears, if you have them, to keep the intensity in the proper range. Long downhill rides will be ineffective.

Stationary exercise bicycles are actually better in many respects than outdoor bikes. They can be used winter or summer in the comfort of your home. Many people read books or watch TV while riding. That way the time goes fast. Again, begin with a low resistance, so that you can complete the entire 20 minutes of exercise. As you toughen your upper legs, you can increase the resistance on the wheel to increase the heart-rate response. The heart-rate techniques discussed earlier in this chapter are especially effective for stationary exercise bicycles. Remember, start at a low level and work up. Try to complete the entire 20 minutes and increase by five minutes a week until you can ride for an hour.

You should be careful to select an exercise bicycle that rides smoothly and is comfortable. Because of the nature of the pedal stroke, exercise bikes need a weighted resistance wheel. A weighted wheel will develop momentum as you ride and will carry the pedals smoothly past the upper and lower positions without so much jerkiness. Bicycles with regular wheels tend to be very jerky as you increase the resistance.

How the resistance is added is also important. Some bikes use a small rubber wheel which is tightened down onto the main wheel. Others use regular center-or side-pull brake mechanisms. The brake mechanisms are better than the wheels for smooth ridings and longevity. However, the best systems use a felt pad on a polished, weighted wheel or a nylon strap around a weighted wheel. These are more expensive but in the long run are probably worth the extra money.

Exercise bicycles that involve movement of the seat and handle bars while riding are not superior to normal bikes. In fact, we prefer to work on flexibility separately. Some people actually get seasick using the moving bikes.

Motorized bikes are difficult to use effectively. You must actively assist the motion of the bike to get a training effect. Otherwise, you're just along for the ride.

Rope Skipping

Rope skipping has become popular among people who exericse. Several physical educators have even claimed that rope skipping is more effective than jogging for developing cardiovascular endurance. However, studies in which the heart rate is controlled show no difference. Both yield about the same effect if the intensity and duration are equalized.

Rope skipping can be done in a limited space such as a backyard or garage. It could also be done in a basement or high family room to avoid the heat or cold associated with activity outdoors. We often take a jumping rope to conventions or when traveling so as to avoid having to run through the busy streets of large cities. Those who are self-conscious about running in view of their neighbors could use rope skipping very effectively.

Little equipment is needed for this activity, and anyone who persists for several weeks can learn the skill. Buy a rope long enough to reach your armpits when you stand on it. Be sure that the rope is fairly heavy so that its momentum will carry it easily over your head as you turn it. A heavy cottonweave or nylon rope will do nicely. Many commercial ropes also work well. Some have bearings, others are woven, some even have digital counters. There is no need for any special counters or other devices. Monitoring the heart rate after each bout of jumping will tell you all you need to know.

It is important to begin slowly and to realize that rope skipping is a very intense activity. You will probably not be able to jump continuously until you have trained for some time. We recommend that you start by jumping with both feet each time the rope hits the ground. Jump for ten or fifteen turns, then walk around for a minute while you get your breath. A few such series will show you how many turns it takes to get your heart rate up to the training level.

After you have jumped for several days, try jumping first on one foot and then the other. Later you will be able to alternate feet in any combination as you turn the rope at a fairly high rate. As you develop skill and endurance, you can increase the number of turns before taking a break. For instance, you may jump 40 to 50 turns, walk around for 20 to 30 seconds, then jump again for the same number, continuing this sequence for 25 to 30 minutes. Be sure to walk, even if you must walk in circles, between sequences. This will insure a positive pumping action from the muscle pump as you relax.

If you don't overdo it during the first few weeks, you will really enjoy this activity. We should warn you that you may experience soreness in the calf muscles and in the shoulder muscles that rotate the rope. Those with back trouble should probably avoid this activity.

Dancing

Aerobic dance (rhythmic, long-duration dancing to develop fitness) is becoming popular in many areas. The proponents of this activity feel that it is much more enjoyable to exercise to music and be creative at the same time than to participate in some "mundane" activity such as jogging. We have wired dancers as they created new and exciting motions to music and the heart rate does respond positively. A training effect will surely occur as long as the principles of intensity, duration, and frequency are followed. We would urge you to check your pulse often at first to insure that your activity is causing the proper heart-rate response. Otherwise, the effectiveness will be decreased.

Minitramp

Bouncing or jogging on a small minitramp can be an effective exercise for losing weight. However, it is important to check your pulse rate from time to time because the springs in the minitramp "help" your exercise and the intensity may be too low to be effective.

Appendix Six
Basics of Nutrition

Our efforts to find nutrition truths have been very frustrating. We have talked with nutritionists and other health professionals, read nutrition texts, and also read some of the recent research. We have formulated ideas about the relationship between diet and health from this mass of confusion, but would have a hard time proving our views with the available scientific data. However, our ideas are very much in keeping with new recommendations made by the American Heart Association and the Senate Select Committee on Nutrition.

We are very confident in our understanding of diet as it pertains to weight control. The low fat, low sugar, high fiber recommendations are in complete harmony with good nutrition for general health. It is beyond the scope of this book to go into much detail about these nutritional principles, but we will give some brief guidelines.

Basic Nutrients

The solid substances (carbohydrates, fats, and proteins) are mechanically broken down in the mouth, churned and kneaded in the stomach, and attacked by enzymes in the small intestines to prepare them for absorption across the cells of the intestinal wall. After they are absorbed they can be used by the cells of the body to carry on their normal functions.

Carbohdyrates. Carbohdyrates are synthesized in plants by the process of photosynthesis. Energy from the sun is used to combine carbon dioxide and water, forming the various plant structures and releasing oxygen in the process.

The most common edible plant structure is starch, a polysaccharide or group of simple sugars found in such foods as seeds, corn, grains, peas, beans, potatoes and roots. Plant starch is the most important source of carbohydrate in the American diet and accounts for about 50 percent of the total carbohydrate we eat.

The large starch molecule cannot be absorbed into the bloodstream so it must be broken down to a simple sugar or monosaccharide by the digestive process. The most prevalent monosaccharide absorbed by the body is glucose, although some fructose and galactose are also absorbed. Fructose is found in fruit, table sugar, and honey and is easily converted to glucose by the body. Two simple sugars form disaccharides and provide another source of simple sugars to the body. For instance, table sugar, or sucrose, is simply glucose and fructose. Sucrose makes up about 25 percent of the total carbohydrate we eat and occurs naturally in most carbohydrate foods especially in beet and cane sugar, sorghum, maple syrup, etc.

The problem with eating large quantities of sucrose is that it contains calories, but no vitamins or minerals. It is often referred to as "empty calorie" food. Another disaccharide, lactose, is found naturally only in milk and is composed of glucose and galactose. Maltose occurs in malt products and germinating cereals and is composed of two glucose molecules. All of these carbohydrates contribute simple sugars for the body to use as energy. These small glucose molecules are carried by the blood to the liver and to the muscles where they are hooked together into a large polysaccharide (much like starch in plants) called glycogen.

Liver glycogen is used as a source of glucose to maintain normal blood sugar levels between meals. When blood sugar begins to drop, the liver releases glucose using a process called glycogenolysis. Muscle glycogen cannot be released, but must be used by the individual muscle for energy.

The main function of carbohydrates is to provide energy for the body, although they are also an important source of vitamins and minerals. The actual production of energy takes place in small capsule-shaped structures called mitochondria that are found in every cell. Training increases their number and efficiency in muscle cells so that more energy can be produced.

Carbohydrates are also essential for the proper functioning of the central nervous system. The brain uses blood glucose almost exclusively, and decreased blood glucose (hypoglycemia) can result in feelings of weakness, hunger, and dizziness.

Carbohydrates are essential for the fat-burning processes as well. If insufficient carbohydrates are burned, fat metabolism cannot continue normally and "ketone bodies" begin to accumulate in the blood. This causes the "acetone" breath sometimes noticed during fasting or as a result of diabetes.

Carbohydrates are also essential in maintaining tissue protein. If carbohydrate intake is severely limited (such as in low-carbohydrate diets), the body has the capacity to break down protein, using a process called gluconeogenesis, to supply blood sugar.

Almost all foods contain some carbohydrates and the typical American diet is about 40 to 50 percent carbohydrate. A recent study showed that a large portion of the carbohydrate intake in overweight females was simple sugars. In fact, the average American eats more than 100 pounds of table sugar each year.

Fats. Fats are long-chain carbon compounds that are generally greasy to the touch and insoluble in water. They are found in both plants and animals, and require bile for proper digestion in the body. Fats are broken down and absorbed as simple fats called fatty acids, and other fat "pieces." Some are carried directly through the portal vein to the liver and the rest are carried as "chylomicrons" in the lymph system until dumped into the bloodstream near the heart. Fats present a special challenge in terms of being carried by the blood because they are hydrophobic, or, in other words, they hate water. Because of this, they are most often packaged with protein to form lipoproteins and in this form are carried to the cells of the body. Lipoproteins (and other such structures) are called compound lipids. Only small amounts of these are found in food, but large numbers are made in the body. Another class of fats is the "derived" lipids. This category includes such lipids as 7-dehydrocholesterol which is the compound found in the fat beneath our skin that produces vitamin D when exposed to sunlight. Another is cholesterol, which plays an important role in the brain, the nervous system, sexual secretions, and digestion.

The primary role of fat is to provide the body with a large store of potential energy for work. Fat is beautifully designed for this purpose, having a little over twice as much potential energy per gram as either protein or carbohydrate. It is easily transported and fits the body nicely in storage, and can be readily converted to energy in the mitochondria.

It is important to realize, however, that large quantities of dietary fat are not needed to provide this storage since excess calories from any source can be changed to fat and stored in the fat cells. Almost all nutritionists and cardiologists feel that the average American diet is too high in fat and recommend a decrease to a more moderate level. Both heart disease and cancer have been linked to high fat intake.

Ingested fats play some essential roles. First, fats carry the lipid soluble vitamins A, D, E, and K. There are also certain "essential fatty acids" that are indispensable to life. These fatty acids are needed for building cell membranes and as constituents for many fundamental chemical compounds. However, our need for them is small, perhaps only 1 to 2 percent of our total calories, and the richest source of them is the vegetable oils!

Fats also serve to cushion and protect vital organs and to provide insulation from the cold. However, it might be better to wear another sweater than to get fat for this purpose because a sweater can be removed when it gets hot.

Protein. Proteins are similar in many respects to both carbohydrates and fats in that they have a carbon skeleton and contain hydrogen and oxygen. However, protein also contains nitrogen and small amounts of sulfur, phosphorus, and iron. Just as glycogen is made up of small simple sugars, proteins are constructed from smaller building blocks called amino acids. There are about 20 amino acids that occur in food proteins, but these 20 small subunits can be arranged in many different forms and lengths providing an almost limitless array of different protein structures in the body. For instance, there are over 100 different enzymes and an enormous variety of hormones and antibodies produced by the body from these amino acids. They are also the principle materials of which the cells of bones, the brain, blood vessels, muscles, nerves, the skin, intestines, and the various glands are made. It is estimated that, in all, the cells of our body produce well over 100,000 different compounds from these few amino acids.

There are nine amino acids that cannot be made by the body and are therefore classified as "essential." If we do not eat foods with enough of the essential amino acids, the inevitable result will be that the body will be unable to produce the proteins it requires for good health. Although there is no difference in the amino acids found in plant and animal proteins, plant proteins are often deficient in one or more of the essential amino acids.

For instance, wheat is low in an amino acid called lysine and beans lack methionine. If your only protein source were either of these vegetables, you would have to eat a rather large quantity to supply enough lysine or methionine. In one study, volunteers were fed a diet that depended on eight slices of bread each meal for total protein. Within a few weeks it was shown that subjects were receiving adequate amino acids even though wheat is known to be deficient in lysine.

A better way to supply essential amino acids from these courses is to combine two "incomplete" proteins that are complementary in terms of their shortage. For instance, eating both wheat and beans allows the protein sources to make up for one another's amino acid deficiencies.

Of course, it might be argued that the problem could be solved by eating only from "high quality" animal protein sources. Although it is true that animal proteins have a better balance of the essential amino acids, they are also one of the primary sources of fat in the diet, and excessive amounts can cause problems in terms of weight control, heart disease, and cancer.

The truth is that protein deficiency is probably the least common of all major nutrient deficiencies in the United States. According to one study, even the lowest income families consume about 2.3 times their average requirements of protein.

If we eat too much protein but too little carbohydrate for our energy needs, much of the protein will lose its nitrogen and be burned as fuel. If we have plenty of calories, excess amino acids can be converted to fat and stored in the fat cells. In both cases, the nitrogen is used by the body to produce other amino acids or is changed to ammonia and excreted. Most of the excretion takes place in the kidneys and can cause an increased urine volume in people who are on a "high protein" reducing diet. This is another reason for the deceptive short-term weight loss associated with this type of diet.

It should be mentioned that the body is thrifty when it comes to protein and conserves many of the amino acids that come from tissue protein and other body chemicals which have been broken down.

This recycling of amino acids is a key factor in determining how much protein we need.

How much protein do we really need? The RDA committee estimated that an average 154-pound man loses about 23 grams of protein a day. This means that about .32 grams of protein per pound of weight needs to be replaced. To be safe, the committee recommended a gram of protein per kilogram (2.2 pounds) per day, or about 56 grams a day for the 154-pound man mentioned above. A person this size eats roughly 2500 calories per day. Since the average diet is about 18 percent protein, he probably gets about 94 grams to replace a real need of about 23 grams.

The RDA committee further concluded that only about 20 percent or 1/2 ounce (12 grams) of the total protein needed to come from the so-called essential amino acids. Obviously, large quantities of animal protein are not needed for good protein nutrition.

Vitamins and Minerals

The metabolic regulatory mechanisms in cells all require small "micronutrients" called vitamins and minerals for proper function.

Vitamins. The importance of vitamins has been recognized since Hippocrates recommended liver to cure night blindness. Scientists have since identified many of these small essential chemicals that are so necessary to health. With few exceptions, humans cannot manufacture vitamins and so must depend on the diet or artificial supplementation.

There are two major classifications for vitamins—those that are water soluble and those that are fat soluble. Table 1 shows the water-soluble vitamins, their best dietary sources, and the major functions of each:

Table 1 — Water-Soluble Vitamins

Vitamin	Best Dietary Source	Major Function
Vit B1 (Thiamine)	Pork, organ meats, whole grains, legumes	Coenzyme or CO_2 removal
Vit B2 (Riboflavin)	In many foods	Carries hydrogen in energy cycle
Niacin	Liver, lean meats, grains, legumes	Coenzyme in energy cycle

Vit B6 (Pyridoxine)	Meats, vegetables, whole grain cereals	Protein metabolism
Pantothenic acid	In many foods	Energy cycle
Folacin	Legumes, green vegetables whole wheat products	Coenzyme - protein
Vit B12	Muscle meats, eggs, dairy food (not in plants)	Nucleic acid metabolism
Biotin	Legumes, vegetables, meats	Coenzyme for fat, carbohydrate, and protein metabolism
Choline	Egg yolks, liver, grains, legumes	Constituent in phospholipids
Vit C	Citrus fruits, tomatoes, salads, green peppers	Collagen synthesis

Because these vitamins are water soluble, they are not stored for long periods in the body and must be replaced regularly. Excessive intakes are not serious because they can be excreted. Table 2 shows the fat-soluble vitamins, their best sources, and what they do.

Table 2 — Fat-Soluble Vitamins

Vitamin	Best Dietary Source	Function
Vit A (Retinol)	Green vegetables, milk, butter, cheese, fortified margarine	Visual pigment
Vit D	Cod liver oil, eggs, dairy products, fortified milk, and margarine	Bone growth
Vit E (Tocopherol)	Seeds, green leafy vegetables, margarine, shortenings	Antioxidant
Vit K (Phylloquinone)	Green leafy vegetables, some in cereals, fruits, meats	Blood clotting

Daily intake of fat-soluble vitamins is not nearly so important because they are stored in the fatty tissue of the body and do not wash out easily. On the other hand, excess quantities can be dangerous for the same reason.

Minerals. Minerals make up approximately 4 percent of the total body weight and can be classified as the "major" minerals and the "trace" minerals. Most of them are found naturally in the waters of rivers, lakes, and oceans; in the topsoil, and root systems of plants and trees; and in the body structure of animals we eat. Table 3 contains the most important minerals, their best dietary source, and their primary functions.

Table 3 - Major Minerals

Mineral	Dietary Source	Function
Calcium	Milk, cheese, dark green vegetables, legumes	Bone and tooth formation
Phosphorus	Milk, cheese, meat, poultry, grains	Bone and tooth formation
Sulfur	Dietary protein	Tissue compound
Potassium	Meat, milk, many fruits	Nerve function, acid-base balance
Chlorine	Salt	Acid-base balance, gastric acid
Sodium	Salt	Acid-base balance, body-water balance,
Magnesium	Whole grains, green leafy vegetables	Activate enzymes, protein synthesis
Iron	Eggs, lean meats, legumes, whole grains, green leafy vegetables	RBC - carries O2 energy system
Fluorine	Water, seafood	Bone structure
Zinc	Many foods	Enzymes - digestion

The major function of minerals is in cellular metabolism where they serve as important parts of enzymes that regulate chemical reactions.

The trace minerals are also important for life. For instance, a lack of a small amount of iodine can result in goiter formation. Such minerals as copper, tin, nickel, selenium, manganese, molybdenum, and chromium are all necessary for life, even if only in minute quantites.

Water. Water is also a necessary nutrient and makes up about 60 percent of total body weight. Chemical reactions in the body take place only in a liquid medium, gases diffuse only across moist membranes; nutrients and wastes are transported in aqueous solutions; and water has tremendous heat-stabilizing qualities. Water also helps give structure and form to the body tissues.

We normally drink about 1200 ml. (just over a quart) of water a day, but this amount may increase dramatically for those who exercise because of the large volume lost in sweat. There is also a small amount of water supplied from foods we eat and from the metabolic processes that produce energy. Many overweight individuals drink very little water.

Appendix Seven
Nutritional Problems from Reducing Diets

The purpose of this appendix is to discuss some of the problems associated with the more typical diets people use. To the best of our knowledge, all reducing diets have encouraged the intake of fewer calories than the body needs to maintain itself. Some diets have allowed all you can eat of certain foods, but because of the low caloric density of the specific food item, fewer total calories have been eaten. Starch blockers allow adequate foods to be eaten but block the breakdown of starch so that fewer total calories are taken into the bloodstream. Low carbohydrate diet proponents have claimed that weight loss will occur while eating huge amounts of protein and fat so long as the carbohydrate calories remain low. Muscle and water will certainly be lost with this type of diet, but whether fat is lost or not is debatable. What usually happens is that the resultant high ketone level artificially suppresses the hunger, the dieter is denied many of his favorite foods, becomes bored with the limited choices and cuts down the total calories.

We have already mentioned the problems produced by inadequate calories (that of stimulating the defense mechanism against starvation and producing vitamin and mineral deficiencies—both of which seem to interfere with weight loss). However, since there are also some more specific dietary problems produced by each type of diet, we will classify diets into several categories and talk about the problems of each.

Balanced Diets

Low-calorie balanced diets have been the most popular of all diets used by health professionals. They produce no better results today than they have in the past. Although the increasingly strong eating drive may be modified by using behavioral modification, most people lose only a very modest amount of weight, if any at all. The starvation defenses are simply too powerful to allow much weight loss. Continued adherence to this type of diet over a very long period might produce the same dangers we see with stricter diets in a short period. Fortunately, most people can't fight against hunger forever and soon return to a normal intake.

Very low-calorie balanced diets usually provide only 300 to 800 calories per day. Various forms have been used for over 30 years. They do have some inherent advantages. Weight loss is rapid and hunger is often suppressed. Some of the diets depend on an extremely low-calorie powdered mixture supposedly containing all of the necessary proteins, carbohydrates, fats, vitamins and minerals necessary for human health. However, recent reports relate these diets to serious illness and possible deaths.

The popular gastric stapling procedures work like a very low-calorie diet, since only limited food intake is possible. We are starting to see unexplained deaths in this group of patients. These deaths are probably due to some vitamin or mineral deficiency or inbalance.

Health professionals have advised repeatedly that these extreme types of diets should be administered and supervised only by experienced physicians. Even then, problems can occur.

Unbalanced Diets

Over the years, many attempts have been made to lose weight with various unbalanced diets. Although diets that were almost exclusively fat or carbohydrate have been used experimentally, few have become popular. One exception is a recent best seller that emphasized fruits. The low-protein levels caused good weight loss, but mainly at the expense of muscle and water. Fortunately, this particular form of craziness seems to be fading.

By far the most popular form of unbalanced diets has been the low carbohydrate diet. This diet achieved an amazing degree of popularity over the past years and even now adversely influences the thinking and eating patterns of many overweight people. This diet has been widely criticized by health authorities and seems to produce the following problems:

- High levels of dietary protein and fats produce high levels of ketones in the bloodstream which tend to change the acid-base balance of the blood.

- Loss of minerals. There is some evidence that high protein diets will leach minerals from the body. Calcium stores in particular may be decreased to very low levels, leading to osteoporosis and easy bone breaking. Other important minerals like zinc, iron, phosphorus and magnesium may also be lost. Vitamins and minerals may also be lacking in these unbalanced diets.
- The high-fat/high-protein food in low carbohydrate diets may be a major contributor to common diseases such as arteriosclerosis, high blood pressure, diabetes, some cancers, constipation and gall bladder disease.
- Low carbohydrate diets seem to interfere with insulin and sugar metabolism. A glucose tolerance test performed on someone with a low carbohydrate diet shows bizarre results with widely fluctuating blood sugars. The high fat and low carbohydrate levels both seem to increase insulin resistance and stimulate fat storage.
- Most people who lose weight with low carbohydrate diets will quickly regain the weight when they return to normal eating, but often retain some food biases against good wholesome foods as a result of their experience.

A new concept of dieting was developed a few years ago called the protein-sparing modified fast. This diet supposedly provided just enough protein to protect against muscle loss as well as loss of all essential vitamins and minerals. Liquid proteins became popular and were widely used until a number of unexplained deaths occurred, then the diet was almost entirely stopped. Refeeding after dieting or overeating during a very low-calorie diet has also been associated with severe illnesses and even death. This may be due to a sudden shifting of various electrolytes in the body.

Every diet has its dangers. The most restrictive should only be used for extreme circumstances under the direct supervision of an experienced physician. The more conservative low-calorie diets are relatively safe, but certainly may produce rather substantial deficiency states if continued long enough. The main problem with any restrictive diet is that the weight-regulating mechanism interprets it as starvation and accordingly resists weight loss and any changes that might help to keep the weight off. Even a good exercise program seems insufficient in compensating for the strong protective mechanisms of the body. The body then remains programmed for fat storage with a high setpoint and various biological changes that conserve energy and protect fat, perhaps attaining even higher fat levels than before the diet began. The ensuing hunger, fatigue, lethargy, weakness, and poor endurance certainly decrease the quality of life. If you are going to use one of these programs for temporary weight loss, it makes more sense to use one that is relatively safe. It makes even more sense to do the right things to reprogram the body to be thinner and to feel energetic, strong, healthy, and be able to eat more food while remaining comfortably stable at a lower weight.

Appendix Eight
How to Get
a Balanced Diet

Many of us eat a diet that lacks some of the basic nutrients for good health. We eat too many prepared and highly refined foods and eat too many meals in fast-food restaurants. Chronic dieters have the added problem of eating too few calories to get proper nutrition.

The daily food records of new patients is alarming. It is not uncommon to see a diet consisting of six bottles of coke, several candy bars and some cookies, donuts or potato chips as the total daily intake. The nutritional highlight of their entire week may be a hamburger, fries, and a shake.

All of us have been taught at least some basics about good nutrition. However, many of us ignore most of this information. This may have something to do with the very permissive era through which we have just passed. The spirit of the seventies seems to have been "if it feels good, do it," or likewise, "if it tastes good, eat it."

Working mothers are often too busy to prepare nutritious meals or teach their children how to cook healthful foods. More and more meals are eaten away from home or are prepared at home from prepackaged convenience sources.

We have a built-in protective drive that attracts us to high-calorie, high-fat, high-sugar foods to ensure adequate nutrients for protection against starvation. Although this drive served us well before refined and convenience foods were so readily available, it can create problems for us today. If we allow ourselves to eat only those things that taste good to our "junk food" appetites, we end up with a diet that will cause fatness and may create many other problems.

Let's analyze the average American diet. The average female eats about 2,000 calories daily; the average male about 3,000 calories. Of these, 40 to 50 percent comes from fats. Refined fats like vegetable oils have few vitamins or minerals. Animal fats have some vitamins and minerals, but very few compared to the total number of calories. In addition, the average American eats about 120 pounds of sugar per year or just over 500 calories per day with no vitamins or minerals. Our diet would then look like this:

	Male	Females
Total calories	3000	2000
Fat calories	1200-1500	800-1000
Sugar calories	600	400
Total fat and sugar calories	1800-2100	1200-1400
Total calories which contain vitamins and minerals	900-1200	600-800

As we have shown in chapter 3, fats and sugars in these quantities will tend to make most of us fat. Obviously, we need to make changes if we as a society hope to become thin and healthy.

Dietary Recommendations

In the 1930s, the Home Economics Research Division of the U.S. Department of Agriculture developed a basic guideline called the Basic Four Food Groups. This was an attempt to encourage people to eat healthy foods to provide all the required nutrients. This guideline will provide your minimum needs, but depending on which foods you add to make up the rest of your required calories, can still cause you to become fat or develop diet-induced diseases (figure A8.1).

In 1977, and again in 1985, the Senate Select Committee on Nutrition made some dietary recommendations to the American public that surely substantiates the need to decrease the level of fat in the diet. According to some nutritionists, these guidelines were a compromise. Apparently, some members of the committee felt that a much lower fat content should be recommended, but because of a concern for the food producers, only modest changes were finally made. In any case, both sets of recommendations will likely provide a nutritious dietary guideline. A reduction of fats and sugars below the 30 percent recommended by the Senate Committee may be even healthier, but this is still controversial. However, there is no controversy about the need to decrease fats and sugars if you have a weight problem. Our experience has shown this change to be essential and we recommend the following:

Fats	10 - 20 percent of total calories
Proteins	10 - 15 percent of total calories
Complex Carbohydrates	65 - 80 percent of total calories
Refined Carbohydrates	0 percent to very small levels

This type of diet is actually fairly easy to follow. Most vegetables, grains and fruits fall within the guidelines, whereas meats and dairy

Figure A8.1   Basic Four Food Groups

Food Group	Serving per day
MILK	
1 c milk, yogurt or calcium	3 for child
Equivalent	4 for adolescent
1 1/2 oz. or 45 gm cheddar	2 for adult
cheese	
1 c pudding;	
1 3/4 c ice cream;	
2 c cottage cheese	
MEAT	2
2 oz cooked, lean meat	
fish, poultry, or Protein	
Equivalent (2 eggs; 2 oz. or	
60 gm cheddar cheese;	
1/2 c cottage cheese;	
1 c dried beans or peas;	
4 tbsp peanut butter; 2 oz. nuts)	
FRUIT-VEGETABLE	4, including
1/2 c cooked or raw	1 from Vitamin C group
1 c raw juice	
GRAIN, whole-grain or enriched	4
1 slice bread; 1 tortilla;	
1 c ready-to-eat cereal;	
1/2 c cooked cereal, rice, pasta,	
grits	

products provide higher protein levels and usually higher fats. By emphasizing vegetables and grains, with some fruit, and only small amounts of meats and dairy products, you will automatically fall within the limits mentioned above.

It is certainly not necessary to count calories, grams of fat, carbohydrates, or proteins. However, there are several ways to estimate fat levels using the food composition section if you wish to. If you merely follow the basic food groups (with minor modification) and add the extra calories entirely from the grains, vegetables and fruits, you can't go too far wrong. Let's now look at each of the basic food groups and recommend some possible modifications.

Milk

Milk provides a great deal of calcium as well as certain other nutrients. However, a large percentage of adults throughout the world cannot drink milk and use few other dairy products. If you emphasize vegetables and grains, you may get plenty of calcium without milk. Some common vegetables such as spinach and beet greens have twice as much calcium per calorie as milk. Unless you are sure of what you are doing, you should still use some milk products. One glass daily would be adequate for adults, with two or three for growing children and adolescents. This should be low fat, either skim or 1 percent. Plain yogurt and low-fat cottage cheese are also good. You should limit most other cheeses since they are very high in fat. Fruit-flavored yogurt is loaded with sugar. Ice cream is high in fat and sugar and should be used rarely and in small amounts.

Meat

You may be surprised to note that we recommend only 3 1/2 to 4 ounces of lean meat a day, a rather large decrease in intake for most of us. If we eat healthy amounts of whole vegetables and grains we can get by with only small amounts of meat. Some vitamins may be a little hard to replace if we completely eliminate meats. For this reason, we don't recommend complete avoidance of meat unless you know a lot about nutrition and can adequately make up for the lack of such vitamins. Be sure to eat only the low-fat meats such as poultry, fish, flank, round or rump cuts of beef. Be careful of meat substitutes like cheddar cheese and peanut butter that are very high in fat.

Fruits and Vegetables

Most fruit tastes good and is fun to eat, but does present a few problems. Because fruit is usually quite low in protein and fats, we can't use it for our major food source. The sugars in fruits are generally in a more simple form than those found in grains and vegetables. Fruit is usually not as satisfying or sustaining as vegetables and cereals, and may be absorbed rather quickly. Processed fruit juices are absorbed more like refined sugars and are not recommended. Many canned or frozen fruits contain added sugar.

Some reducing diets have emphasized fruit and fruit juices. A recent fad diet advocated eating only fruit for several weeks at a time. These programs promote protein and muscle loss and are, of course, not helpful. We wish to put fruit in its proper perspective. It has no magical properties for fat loss. As part of a balanced diet with abundant vegetables and grain products, several fruit servings a day are highly recommended.

Most vegetables have an excellent blend of protein, fat, and carbohydrates as well as being high in vitamins and minerals. They also have a very low caloric density. For example, you would need to eat about 40 pounds of lettuce per day to get 2000 calories of food energy. Even the highest caloric density vegetables like potatoes would require over seven pounds to give you 2000 calories. This low caloric density feature is useful because you get lots of chewing, tasting and stomach filling with vegetables, which helps to produce satiety. It can also help dilute the influence of high caloric foods. However, vegetables may be relatively unsatisfying unless mixed with more calorically dense foods. You simply couldn't eat the 40 pounds or so of lettuce to provide your daily caloric needs.

Vegetables contain fiber and their nutrients are complex so that digestion and absorption are slowed. This provides a steady flow of nutrients into the blood for a number of hours and keeps insulin levels low, which in turn reduces the need for stress hormones to counteract rapid sugar drops associated with the intake of refined sugar.

Many overweight people, especially overweight children, eat too few vegetables. Without vegetables in the diet, food is generally high in caloric density and there are usually more fats and sugars present. It is also easier to develop vitamin and mineral deficiencies. Any of these factors may help to move the setpoint higher.

Eating vegetables is almost a must to become comfortably reprogrammed at a lower weight level. Even if you already enjoy vegetables, you may find it useful to increase their proportion in your diet.

Many children dislike vegetables and must develop a taste for them. The problem may be due to an acquired taste for sweets which makes vegetables seem bland by comparison. Some adults avoid vegetables as a form of continued rebellion against parents who forced vegetables on them when they were young.

The following suggestions may be helpful in developing a taste for vegetables, and for teaching children to like vegetables too.

- Greatly reduce refined carbohydrates, artificial sweeteners and salt in your diet. After a week or so, your taste will change and you will enjoy many foods which formerly were too bland, bitter, or sour for your taste.
- Try eating and serving vegetables raw. Cauliflower, cabbage, broccoli, beans, peas, zucchini, turnips and potatoes which are usually cooked can all be very enjoyable when eaten raw. Most of us prefer the old standards like tomatoes, carrots, celery and cucumbers when served raw. You can use a low-fat vegetable dip made from yogurt or cottage cheese, but after a while you can reduce the amount of dip and gradually learn to enjoy the vegetable taste by itself.
- Introduce sweet vegetables such as potatoes, corn, peas, beans, and raw carrots first.
- Choose very fresh, high-quality vegetables. Freshly picked vegetables are much better tasting than those that have been picked several days before or shipped long distances.

Breads and Cereals

Grains are the staple food in the diet of most people in the world. However, in America we have been taught that bread, rice, cereals, and starchy vegetables are fattening and have switched to meat, cheddar cheese and other problem foods instead.

We recommend that you make grain products a major part of your diet. For many people a slice of whole wheat bread provides a more satisfying and sustaining snack than fruits and vegetables. Bread can also be added as a part of a good light breakfast or lunch. Brown rice is also an ideal food and should be frequently eaten as a major part of a nutritious diet. You could certainly eat grain more often than the four servings suggested in the basic food groups. Ten servings would be no problem for most people once a good exercise program has raised the metabolic rate to higher levels and the set-point has moved downward.

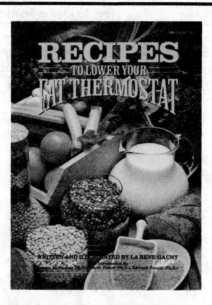

RECIPES TO LOWER YOUR FAT THERMOSTAT is a companion to **HOW TO LOWER YOUR FAT THERMOSTAT**. It provides a rainbow of recipes to make lowering your setpoint deliciously easy. Here are some of the highlights from the cookbook:

- Make it easy to give your family well balanced, satisfying meals that they will love while you lose weight.
- Use the many helpful suggestions for hearty brown-bag lunches, traveling and eating out.
- Enjoy a variety of breakfast, lunch and dinner menus.
- Learn secrets to change your own recipes into setpoint-lowering recipes.
- Make good goodies for snacks, desserts, and for guests that you can enjoy along with everyone else.
- Make your family healthier foods that reduce the risk of heart attacks, cancer and other serious diseases.
- Add variety, interest and excitement to your meals with over 400 tasty recipes to put an end to boredom and ho-hum meals.
- Every recipe gives the RCU, FU, calorie, protein, fat, carbohydrate and sodium count.

RECIPES TO LOWER YOUR FAT THERMOSTAT is a top quality book with over 430 pages and plenty of full-color photographs. It is available in most bookstores. If you can't locate a copy you can obtain it directly from the publisher.

Send a check for $14.95 plus $2.00 for shipping and handling, a total of $16.95, to:

RECIPES
VITALITY HOUSE INTERNATIONAL, INC.
1675 North Freedom Blvd. 11-C
Provo, Utah 84604

Appendix Nine
Recipes and Food Use Guidelines

In this section we present ideas about food preparation that fit in well with the suggested dietary management principles. Rather than simply giving a list of recipes, we will include some basic information about foods.

Wheat

Wheat is an outstanding food because it has an ideal blend of protein, complex carbohydrate and fat (12 to 16 percent protein, 3 to 5 percent fat and 81 to 85 percent complex carbohydrate). It lacks some essential vitamins and minerals and thus can't provide all of our needs, but can be used as a major food source. Unfortunately, the vast majority of wheat used in the modern world has been highly refined. This process involves breaking the wheat down into very small particles, throwing away the bran and the wheat germ, and keeping the starch, thus wasting the fiber and many of the vitamins and minerals. It is now well known that reduced fiber in the diet contributes to bowel cancer, gall bladder disease and constipation.

White flour stores well because most organisms can't live on it. That should tell us something about its value as human food. Also, since the wheat germ part is removed, there are no oils to go rancid. However, whole wheat flour spoils rather quickly and begins to lose nutrients. Therefore, it needs to be purchased fresh or ground fresh frequently. Excess flour should be stored in a freezer. If you use whole wheat regularly, you will want to purchase a small wheat grinder.

Wheat kernels can be chewed directly as a snack. It can also be eaten as puffed wheat either as a snack or as breakfast food. Whole wheat can be made into a delicious porridge. A large quantity can be cooked, kept in the refrigerator, then quickly warmed in the microwave or on the stove for a fast, nutritious breakfast.

Whole wheat can be used in making breads, pancakes, waffle mixes, and bran muffins. Although cookies and cakes are not ideal foods, the nutritional quality can be greatly enhances by using whole wheat flour and substituting honey as shown in the recipes in this section.

People often experience some bowel cramping, extra gas, loose bowel movements or diarrhea when they being to eat more wheat. However, thebowelgradually adjusts to the new input and the symptoms usually go away. You may wish to dilute the whole wheat half and half with white flour until your body adjusts.

Bagels

1 pkg active dry yeast	1 tsp salt
1 C warm water (105-115)	2 3/4 C whole wheat flour
1 tsp honey	2 qts water

Dissolve yeast in 1 cup warm water in large mixing bowl. Stir in honey, salt and 1 1/4 cup flour. Beat until smooth. Stir in remaining flour. Knead on lightly floured surface for 10 minutes or until smooth and elastic. Spray bowl with non-stick spray; place in bowl. Cover, let rise in warm place until doubled (about 15 minutes-dough is ready if an indentation remains when touched). Punch down dough; divide into 8 equal portions. Shape each piece into a smooth ball; punch hole in center and pull gently to enlarge hole and make uniform shape. Let rise 20 minutes. Heat oven to 375 degrees. Heat two quarts water to boiling in large kettle. Reduce heat; add 4 bagels. Simmer 7 minutes, turning once. Drain on kitchen towel. Repeat with remaining bagels. Bake on greased baking sheet until bagels are golden brown, 30-35 minutes.

Yield: 8 servings

	RCU	FU	CAL	%F	P	F	C	Na
per serving	0	0	16	4	1	T	3	15

Whole Wheat Pancakes - J.N.

Mix together:	1 1/2 C whole wheat flour
	1/4 tsp salt
	1 3/4 tsp baking soda
Add:	3/4 C buttermilk
	3/4 C apple juice
Fold in:	2 egg whites (beaten) and 1 whole egg

Yield: 12 pancakes

	RCU	FU	CAL	%F	P	F	C	Na
per pancake	0	0	64	10	3	1	12	213

100% Whole Wheat Bread (no oil) - J.N.

Put into mixing bowl:	2 C warm water
	2 T yeast
Blend together in blender:	2 C unsweetened pineapple juice
	4 - 5 raw apples, cored but not peeled
Combine and add to above:	10 1/2 - 11 cups whole wheat flour
	1 C powdered milk
	2 tsp salt
	(only 1 tsp after 3 or 4 batches)

Put into four loaf pans - let rise (not quite double). Bake 45 min. at 350 degrees.

Yield: 24 slices

	RCU	FU	CAL	%F	P	F	C	Na
per slice	0	0	52	4	2	T	11	58

Cracked Wheat Cereal - J.N.

1 cup whole wheat placed in blender - blend at high speed 40 seconds. Stir into 3 cups boiling water - turn off heat and let set 15 minutes. Add 1/8 teaspoon maple flavoring if desired. Season with raisins and fruit - bananas, peaches, etc.

Yield: 4 servings

	RCU	FU	CAL	%F	P	F	C	Na
per serving	0	0	22	5	1	T	5	T

Grape Nut Whole Wheat Muffins - J.N.

Combine in mixing bowl:	1 C Grape Nuts
	3/4 C apple juice
	1/4 C milk
	1 C whole wheat flour
	1/4 tsp salt
	2 tsp baking powder
Add and beat hard one minute:	2 egg whites
Add and beat:	1/2 C raisins
	1/2 C dates

Spoon into muffin pan and bake at 400 degrees for 20 minutes.

Yield: 12 muffins

	RCU	FU	CAL	%F	P	F	C	Na
per muffin	1	T	139	16	3	3	26	63

Rice

Rice is the most commonly used cereal product throughout the world and is perhaps the most commonly known food of any type. It consists of approximately 8 percent protein, 5 percent fat, and 87 percent complex carbohydrate. Used in conjunction with other foods which are higher in protein content, and that contain the vitamins and minerals lacking in rice, it can be an ideal food. Most of us should probably increase the amount of rice in our diets.

Several forms of rice are available. Brown rice is rice that has had the hull removed but retains most of the bran and germ. White or polished rice has both the bran and germ removed. Some white rice has been pre-cooked, is very quick to prepare and may be referred to as minute or instant rice. Parboiled rice has been partly cooked before the hull and bran are removed, which tends to increase the nutrient content. A comparison of the vitamin and mineral content of brown rice compared to white rice if very revealing. Brown rice has at least twice the nutrient content for most nutrients, and up to six times the nutrient level of some vitamins and minerals. Fiber content is also about three times higher in brown rice.

Not only does brown rice have better nutrient properties, it also has a nice nutty flavor and is much more sustaining than white rice. Parboiled rice is also better than white rice since it has better nutrient content but has many of the cooking properties of white rice.

Rice can be used in any situation where potatoes might be used. It can also be topped with gravy or any other topping used for potatoes or it can be made more interesting by adding a little wild rice or a few vegetables to make Chinese fried rice as a one-dish meal or with some other food. A Japanese dish, Sukiyaki, can be used on top of rice. It is very easy to develop your own rice casserole recipes. Start with rice; add a small amount of meat (either leftover cooked meat or freshly cooked). Add a liquid or binder, some vegetables, and herbs or spices if desired. Add the amounts that you desire of meat and vegetables and rice. The liquid could be soups, broth, gravy, juices or water. The amount to be used would be the amount needed to cook the rice according to rice directions) plus 1/2 to 1 cup depending on the amount of meat and vegetables added. Add herbs and spices carefully to begin with; allow for some cooking time and taste. Plain cooked rice or rice with raisins makes a great dessert. A custard rice pudding, while having some sugar, is still better than most desserts.

Spanish Rice

1 med onion diced	1/2 lb lean ground beef
1 sm green pepper, diced	16 oz can of tomatoes, pureed
1/2 C rice (not minute rice)	1 bay leaf
1 whole clove	1/8 tsp crunched red pepper

Place 1 teaspoon oil in kettle and saute onions until soft, add ground beef and brown. Drain fat from meat, then add all the other ingredients. Bring to a boil, stir and turn the heat down. Simmer, stirring often to prevent sticking, 30 minutes or until rice is tender.

Yield: 4 servings

	RCU	FU	CAL	%F	P	F	C	Na
per serving	0	1	296	21	20	7	31	35

Sukiyaki

This is an adaptation of a Japanese dish to serve over rice. There are many possibilities for meats and vegetables in this recipe, however, you should probably use only one kind of meat and 4 to 6 kinds of vegetables at any one time.

Use 1/3 to 1/2 pound of thinly sliced raw meat: pork, chicken, beef or lamb. Use any combination of sliced onions, chunks of green onions, leeks, carrots sliced on the diagonal, celery sliced on the diagonal, strips of cabbage or Chinese cabbage, pieces of broccoli, bean sprouts, snow peas, zucchini sliced diagonally or strips, water chestnuts, green pepper chunks, mushroom slices or pieces, cauliflower pieces, green bean pieces (1 1/2 inch), or bamboo shoots. Can be flavored with soy sauce.

Sukiyaki is prepared in the traditional Oriental way with the vegetables being cooked only until heated through but still crisp. For an interesting effect, it can be cooked right at the table. It is a good idea to prepare and slice all the ingredients and gather them together in the cooking area, set the table, and have the rice cooked before you begin the cooking. Add a small amount of oil or degreased chicken broth to a hot wok or frying pan (only use enough to keep ingredients from sticking). Stir-fry onions and meat slices until meat is just browned. Then begin to add the vegetables starting with those that take the longest to cook (carrots, beans, cauliflower, mushrooms zucchini, celery, broccoli, snow peas). Stir-fry carefully. Then add those that just need to be heated through (cabbage, Chinese cabbage, water chestnuts, bamboo shoots, green pepper, bean sprouts). Add soy sauce to taste (if you use a very strong soy sauce, you may wish to add a little water to make more sauce). You may wish to season with a little salt and pepper and serve quickly over hot rice with toasted sesame seeds.

Yield: 4 servings

	RCU	FU	CAL	%F	P	F	C	Na
per serving	0	0	334	12	21	5	56	170

Shrimp Curry

1 T butter

1/2 C chopped green pepper

2 C plain yogart

2 tsp lemon juice

1/2 tsp ground ginger

3 cups or less cleaned, cooked or canned shrimp

2 cloves garlic minced (or garlic salt depending on taste)

1/2 C chopped onion

1/2 C diced apple, opt

2 to 3 tsp curry powder

1/2 tsp salt

dash chili powder

In saucepan melt butter. Add onions, apples and garlic. Cook until tender but not brown. Add green pepper, yogurt and all other ingredients and a dash of black pepper. Cook over low heat, stirring constantly until heated through (do not boil). Care must be taken to use low heat and constant stirring or this will curdle. Serve over hot cooked rice. Can be served with condiment such as coconut, chopped peanuts, raisins, or chutney. Chicken could be substituted in the form of diced cooked chicken breast.

Yield: 4 servings

	RCU	FU	CAL	%F	P	F	C	Na
per serving	0	1	418	17	36	8	50	340

Beef Curry

1/2 lb beef	1/2 C onion chunks
2 to 3 tsp curry	1/2 tsp ginger
bay leaf	
1 C fresh green beans cut in 1" pieces	

Use chuck, round roast or stewing meat and slice thin in 1" long pieces discarding all visible fat. Brown meat in heavy kettle until there are lots of browned juices. Add water (about 3 or 4 cups) and stew with bay leaf for about 2 hours. Add onions, curry powder, and ginger and cook until onions are just transparent. Add the beans and serve when the beans are heated through but still slightly crisp. Serve over hot cooked rice.

Yield: 4 servings

	RCU	FU	CAL	%F	P	F	C	Na
per serving	0	1	353	25	21	8	44	34

Potatoes

Potatoes are an excellent food (about 11 percent protein, 1 percent fat and 88 percent carbohydrate). They are also an excellent source of potassium and vitamin C and contain other vitamins and minerals as well. Contrary to the diet philosophies of recent years, potatoes are good for you and can be used as a major part of a healthful diet.

Perhaps the major problem with potatoes is that they are often prepared by adding fat. For instance, deep-fat frying triples the calories; whereas, making them into potato chips increases the calories by a factor of ten. The value of baked potatoes are decreased by adding butter and/or sour cream, and mashed potatoes often seem to be eaten with butter and high-fat gravy.

Surprisingly, potatoes taste okay without any topping once you develop the taste. Until then, decrease the among of butter, sour cream or gravy you use. Cook hash browns in a teflon pan with a non-stick spray and use potatoes as the staple item in soup or as the major ingredient in a casserole.

Layered Potato Casserole

Spray a 1 1/2 - 2 quart casserole dish with non-stick spray. In the bottom, place 1 small sliced onion, one layer. On top add a layer of 1/2 pound of very lean ground beef. 3 large sliced potatoes make the next layer. Canned or frozen 10 ounce package of corn on top of the potatoes and then a can of cream of mushroom soup (condensed) over the top. Bake covered in a 375 degree oven for 1 to 1 1/2 hours until the potatoes are tender.

Yield: 6 servings

	RCU	FU	CAL	%F	P	F	C	Na
per serving	0	0	33	20	2	T	5	48

Potato and Hamburger Casserole

1/2 lb. lean hamburger
1/2 C sliced celery, carrots etc.
1 can tomato soup

1/2 C chopped onion
10 oz. pkg. frozen peas
mashed potatoes

Saute onions and cook hamburger in a heavy pan or frying pan, drain hamburger. Add tomato soup, celery, carrots, peas. heat through. Put this mixture in the bottom of casserole dish, cover with mashed potatoes and sprinkle the top with a small amount of parmesan cheese and pepper. Bake at 350 degrees oven for 1 hour. (See page 135)

Yield: 4 servings

	RCU	FU	CAL	%F	P	F	C	Na
per serving	0	1	324	27	23	10	30	490

Baked potatoes can be topped with a variety of meat and vegetable mixtures to make a good main meal. This idea is an adaptation of the fast-food potato outlets often found in shopping centers and can be very low-calorie and delicious.

Beans

There are several different forms of beans. Stringless, wax, green or snap beans are eaten with the bean pods in an immature state and are similar to other garden vegetables. Kidney, pinto or navy beans are the seed portion and are dried to about 10 percent water content. Lima beans are also seeds but are eaten in the immature form much like peas.

Bean in this section refers to the various dried seed forms. These beans form a staple part of the diet for many areas of the world, especially Central and South America. They are high in protein (26 percent), low in fat (4 percent) and are about 70 percent complex carbohydrate. They can be used as a meat substitute, but should be eaten with another type of protein to make a complete protein. Eating beans with rice, corn, wheat products, cheese or meat can enhance their protein quality.

Beans can be cooked, baked or put into a soup. They are also the major ingredient in chili. Refried beans can serve as the basis for many types of meals. In addition to the included recipes, Mexican food cookbooks may contain many ideas for using beans as a nutritious, delicious food substance.

Mexican Pinto Beans Spice Mix- J.N.

5 tsp cumin	5 T dried minced onions
5 tsp chili powder	5 T dried minced garlic
2 1/2 tsp pepper	2 1/2 tsp salt

Combine spices and store in covered bottle. For every 1 cup of beans use 3 tablespoons mix. Use within 2 months.

	RCU	FU	CAL	%F	P	F	C	Na
per Tbls	0	0	7	T	T	T	1	301

Mexican Pinto Beans -M.B.

1 C pinto beans   4 C water
3 T Mexican Pinto Bean Spice Mix

Boil beans in water for 10 minutes. Simmer for 3 hours. Add seasoning mix and cook for 20 minutes before serving.

Yield: 6 servings

	RCU	FU	CAL	%F	P	F	C	Na
per serving	0	0	136	3	7	T	25	158

Refried Beans (bland)

1 lb. dried pinto or pink beans   5 C water
1or 2 medium onions (optional)   salt to taste

Thoroughly wash and drain beans. Place beans in water with onions
either to soak overnight or bring to a boil, cover, remove from heat
and let stand for 1 hour. Return to heat, bring to a boil and cover;
simmer about 3 hours or until beans are tender and mash readily.
You may need to add more water so watch carefully. Mash with
potato masher or in mixer. More water may be needed to bring to the
consistency desired. Serve hot or reheat. Can be used in or with
tacos, enchiladas, burritos, nachos or as a dip. A very good meatless
meal can be made using refried beans and taco accompaniments
(lettuce, cheese, sliced tomatoes, salsa) eaten with taco chips made
from corn tortillas cut in wedges and baked in the oven until crisp.

Yield: 8 servings

	RCU	FU	CAL	%F	P	F	C	Na
per serving	0	0	205	2	13	T	39	245

Refried Beans (spicy) - M.B.

1 recipe Mexican Pinto Beans

Heat heavy frying pan. Add cooked, mashed pinto beans. Stir until any excess water has cooked off and beans have become creamy with a light color. This may be served alone or with rice.

Yield: 6 servings

	RCU	FU	CAL	%F	P	F	C	Na
per serving	0	0	136	3	7	T	25	158

Tomatoes

Tomatoes have about 20 percent protein and are a very good source of vitamin C, vitamin A and potassium. They can be used as a side dish served either fresh or stewed. They can form the basic ingredient for many dishes and can lower the caloric value of foods that use a cream base. Tomatoes can be used in soups, toppings for potatoes or rice, in chili, in spaghetti sauce, or in many other dishes. As a spaghetti sauce, it can be used over cooked cauliflower, whole wheat spaghetti, rice or potatoes.

See Soups, Chili in bean section.

Spaghetti Sauce   (over whole wheat spaghetti)

1/2 lb. lean hamburger
16 oz. can tomatoes pureed
1 can sliced mushrooms & juice
1 T Lawry's Spaghetti Sauce Seasoning mix
parsley, oregano, sweet basil

7 1/2 oz. can tomato sauce
2 T flour
pepper

Brown and crumble hamburger in a large frying pan (drain and pat excess fat). Add flour and stir into hamburger. Return to heat and add tomato sauce, pureed tomatoes, canned mushrooms and juice and seasonings to taste. Simmer for 1/2 hour to 1 hour and serve

over cooked whole wheat spaghetti.   Tastes very good over cauliflower as well.

Yield: 8 servings

	RCU	FU	CAL	%F	P	F	C	Na
per serving	0	T	158	21	12	4	15	154

with cauliflower instead of spaghetti noodles

	RCU	FU	CAL	%F	P	F	C	Na
per serving	0	0	128	23	11	3	10	160

Lasagna

Lasagna, because of all the cheese, is not particularly low calorie;
however, this recipe has less fat than some.

2% mozzarella cheese
Ricotta or low-fat cottage cheese
6 to 8 whole wheat lasagna noodles

parmesan cheese
1 recipe Spaghetti Sauce

Spray 1 1/2 to 2 quart casserole dish with non-stick spray. Put a
layer of sauce in the bottom, a layer of sliced mozzarella, then cottage cheese and noodles. Finally, cover with sauce and a sprinkle of
parmesan cheese. Bake in 350 degree oven for 1 hour. To lower the
fat content, use only a small amount of cheese.

Yield: 6 servings

	RCU	FU	CAL	%F	P	F	C	NA
per serving	2	T	289	18	18	6	35	208

Soups

Soups and stews can provide a very effective way to incorporate the management principles into your diet. They are easy to prepare, inexpensive, very satisfying and can make an entire meal.

For a main meal, soup should contain some basic staple foods such as potatoes, rice, barley, beans, peas, lentils or even tomatoes. They can be served with a small amount of meat or meatless. Avoid cream-based soups and excessive use of noodles because of the extra calories and fat content. Commercially canned soups may have sweeteners added and will not taste as good as homemade, but they are easy to use and can be a good product if chosen carefully.

Keep the water you drain off cooked vegetables (including all canned, fresh and frozen vegetables) to use as the stock for your next soup. This adds a great deal of variety to the flavor and will improve the nutritional content.

Brunswick Stew - J.N.

1 frying chicken, cup up	1 C water

Cover chicken with water in dutch oven, cook 30 to 40 minutes until chicken is tender, cook, debone, and break into pieces.

17 oz can whole kernel corn	1 C sliced onion
1 can (1 lb.) tomatoes	2 cloves garlic, crushed
1 pkg (10 oz.) frozen lima beans	1/4 tsp salt
1 chicken bouillon cube	1/4 tsp pepper
dash cayenne pepper, optional	

Add to broth and cook 30 minutes. Make a past with 3 tablespoon flour and 3 tablespoon milk. Add to stew, stir until slightly thickened. Add meat.

Yield: 8 servings

	RCU	FU	CAL	%F	P	F	C	NA
per serving	0	0	21	10	2	T	2	20

Turkey Vegetable and Noodle soup - J.N.

2 quarts turkey broth
1 C carrots, sliced
1/4 C chopped onion
10 oz pkg. frozen baby lima beans
2 C turkey meat, cut up
1 C uncooked noodles (whole wheat noodles - buy at health
food stores)

1 C potatoes, cubed
1 C celery, sliced
1/4 tsp salt
dash pepper

Add vegetables to turkey broth along with salt, pepper and noodles. Simmer 30 minutes or until tender. Add turkey meat, heat through and serve.

Yield: 6 servings

	RCU	FU	CAL	%F	P	F	C	NA
per serving	T	0	157	12	20	2	23	687

Meats

The amount of fat in meat varies tremendously from one type of meat to another. Most fish and fowl are low in fat as are some cuts of beef (flank, round and rump). Avoid the extremely fat meats such as ham, bacon, hot dogs, and lunch meats. Check the food guideline in appendix 13 for fat content before you buy. In chicken and turkey, the white meat is lower in fat than the dark and in both the skin is high in fat.

All meats are leaner when cooked properly. Use a Teflon or non-stick pan and use vegetable oil spray when frying. Baking, broiling, barbecuing, or using a microwave oven are even better ways of cooking to reduce fats. Alter recipes so that meats are a condiment or smaller portion of the dish rather than being the main entree.

See Sukiyaki, Chili, Spanish Rice recipes.

Oven Fried Chicken

Spray a cookie sheet with non-stick spray. Place raw chicken pieces on the pan (either straight breasts, thighs, legs or combinations, or a whole chicken cut up in usual fryer pieces). Sprinkle with pepper and Lawry's Pinch of Herbs. Place in 375 degree oven and cook for 45 to 60 minutes, depending on the size of the pieces.

Yield: 10 servings

	RCU	FU	CAL	%F	P	F	C	NA
per serving	0	0	82	25	14	2	0	40

Creole

1/2 lb meat (hamburger, cooked diced chicken, shrimp or other seafood)

1/2 C diced onion	1/2 C diced green pepper
1/2 C sliced celery	16 oz can tomatoes, pureed
sprinkle of dried, crushed red pepper	1/4 tsp chili powder

In heavy kettle or frying pan saute onions in 1 teaspoon oil until transparent. Add meat. If you use hamburger, cook thoroughly, drain off oil and pat with paper towel to eliminate fat. Add tomatoes, green pepper, celery and spices and cook until everything is hot, but celery and green peppers are still slightly crisp. Serve over hot cooked rice or baked potato.

Yield: 4 servings

with hamburger

	RCU	FU	CAL	%F	P	F	C	NA
per serving	0	1	364	20	21	8	47	206

with chicken

	RCU	FU	CAL	%F	P	F	C	NA
per serving	0	0	273	9	16	3	47	201

with shrimp

	RCU	FU	CAL	%F	P	F	C	NA
per serving	0	0	281	7	19	2	47	179

Barbecue Chicken - J.N.

2 chickens - skinned and cut up. Arrange in a shallow baking dish (9 x 13). Place 2 onions cut in rings on chicken (may use 2 teaspoon dried onion). Pour sauce over chicken, cover and bake 1½ hours at 350 degrees; uncover and bake 10 minutes more.

Sauce:

3/4 C catsup
3/4 C water
2 T vinegar
1/4 tsp pepper

1 tsp chili powder
1/2 tsp salt
1 tsp paprika
1 1/2 T Worchestershire sauce

Use cooked sauce over baked potatoes or for French dip chicken sandwiches.

Yield: 20 servings

	RCU	FU	CAL	%F	P	F	C	NA
per serving	0	0	107	13	14	2	7	147

Chicken and Broccoli Casserole

1 C cooked diced chicken or turkey
1/2 C sliced celery (not too fine)
1 C broccoli cut in small pieces
1 C parboiled or brown rice

1/2 C diced onion
1/2 C sliced mushrooms
2 C water or chicken broth
1 can cream of mushroom soup

Add all ingredients except broccoli. Stir well. Bake in 350 degree oven in covered casserole dish for 45 minutes or until rice is almost cooked, stir in broccoli and cook for another 15 minutes. It is extra special if you add toasted slivered almonds to the top of the casserole. Leave uncovered in oven for 5 minutes, then serve.

Yield: 6 servings

	RCU	FU	CAL	%F	P	F	C	NA
per serving	0	T	213	15	13	2	32	429

Quick Meal Ideas

One of the major eating problems of the modern world is that many people don't have time to cook a quality meal. With the increase in the number of working mothers, the affluence of society and the ready availability of fast-foods, an increasing number of meals are eaten out. Nearly two-thirds of all meals eaten in America are eaten away from home. We think it is difficult to eat out that often and consistently provide proper nutrition.

People should develop quick meal ideas that can be eaten soon after returning from work. This would decrease the problem of snacking while waiting for a meal, although at times snacking can be quite appropriate. Many modern homes have a time-cooking feature on the oven so that a meal can be cooked just prior to your arrival home. Crock pots can also be used to have a meal completed when you return from work.

Microwave cooking is so fast that you can prepare a full meal in only minutes. Some meals can be prepared in advance (on the weekend), put in the freezer and then used during the week. "TV-type dinners" are excellent if a more suitable ratio of vegetables to meat is used than is commercially available. These dinners can be quickly warmed upon returning home.

With refrigeration, many foods can be prepared in bulk and used two or more times during the week. A casserole or soup provides a good meal a day or two later with little preparation effort.

Most commercially prepared foods are too salty, often have high sugar and/or fat levels, and may be much more expensive than foods that you prepare yourself. However, by reading labels and being selective, you may find convenience foods that are quite acceptable.

There are many recipe books available for crock pot cooking, microwave cooking, and other quick food ideas. Check for those food recipes which conform to the prescribed management principles. Following are a few ideas:

Dressings and Dip Recipes

Zesty Dressing - J.N.

1 T cornstarch   1/2 tsp dry mustard

Mix and add 1 cup cold water.
Cook, stirring constantly until thick, cool.

Add:

1/4 C vinegar   1/4 C catsup
1/2 tsp paprika   1/2 tsp horseradish, opt
1/2 tsp Worchestershire sauce   dash of salt

Beat until smooth. Add 1 clove garlic halved, cover, store in refrigerator.   Shake well before using.

	RCU	FU	CAL	%F	P	F	C	NA
per Tbls	0	0	6	9	T	T	2	3

Russian Dressing

2 sm carrots, thinly sliced
1/2 med tomato
2 T freshly squeezed lemon juice
1/4 C onion, finely chopped

1/2 C water
1/2 C salad vinegar
1 tsp paprika

Simmer carrots in water until tender. Puree the tomato in blender. Add cooked carrots and water, blend with remaining ingredients until smooth. Chill.

	RCU	FU	CAL	%F	P	F	C	NA
per Tbls	0	0	8	T	T	T	1	5

French Dressing

1 C cooked yams, peeled and mashed
1/2 C rice vinegar
1 T apple juice concentrate
2 T lemon juice
dash cayenne pepper
1/2 tsp dry mustard

1/4 tsp onion powder
3/4 C water
1 T soy sauce
1/4 tsp garlic powder
2 T salt-free tomato paste

Mix the liquid ingredients and set aside; mix the dry spices. Gradually add a little of each to yams in blender and blend until smooth.

Yield: 20 tablespoons

	RCU	FU	CAL	%F	P	F	C	NA
per Tbls	0	0	13	3	T	T	3	68

Tomato Dressing - J.N.

1 8-oz. can tomato sauce
1 tsp onion juice
1/4 tsp basil
1 tsp Worchestershire sauce

1 T tarragon vinegar
1/4 tsp dillweed
dash of salt and pepper

Cover and shake well. Chill.

	RCU	FU	CAL	%F	P	F	C	NA
per Tbls	0	0	6	T	T	T	1	3

Dessert Ideas

Dessert can be a major problem for many people. Traditional desserts like cake, pie, ice cream, and puddings are loaded with sugar and fat, are high in calories, and usually encourage overeating. By serving them less often, keeping the size of the serving small, and "saving room" for them so that you do not eat
beyond satiety, you can reduce the harmful effects. Another helpful technique is to change the recipes to improve the quality of the dessert, or use dessert ideas that are inherently healthier.

Some of these items are not particularly healthful, nor do they follow the guidelines very closely. They are, however, an improvement over conventional desserts. Hopefully, you will use your new understanding of the prescribed principles to make wise choices.

Rice Pudding

2 egg whites
1 1/2 C cooked rice
1/4 C raisins
cinnamon

1/4 C honey
2 C skim or 1% milk
1 tsp vanilla

Beat eggs, add milk and honey and beat well. Pour into baking dishes and add rice, vanilla and raisins. Sprinkle a little cinnamon on top and bake in 325 degree oven for 25 minutes. Stir and add more cinnamon if desired. Continue baking for 20 to 25 minutes longer. Serve warm or chilled.

Yield: 4 servings

	RCU	FU	CAL	%F	P	F	C	NA
per serving	3	0	210	T	8	T	45	86

Baked Apples

4 apples

Wash, core and halve apples. Place in a glass baking dish; put 1/4 to 1/2 teaspoon honey in each cavity. Cover the bottom of the dish with water from 1/8- to 1/4- inch depth. Sprinkle the apples with nutmeg and/or cinnamon. Cook covered in oven at 400 degrees until apples are tender (30 to 60 minutes).

Yield: 4 apples

	RCU	FU	CAL	%F	P	F	C	NA
per apple	T	0	91	T	T	T	23	1

Bottle Fruit Cake - Kay Cavender
(serves 12)

1 quart unsweetened fruit mixed in blender, juice and all

Add: 1 egg
                                                    3 tsp soda
and set aside.

Mix together:

1 C bottled fruit drained   1 C apple juice
                                                    (unsweetened) and
                                                    mashed (or pureed in1
                                                    tsp salt blender)
1 tsp cloves   4 C whole wheat flour
1 tsp nutmeg   2 1/2 tsp cinnamon

Mix well in mixer, add fruit and egg mixture. Mix well. Add raisins
and dates as desired. Bake 45 minutes at 350 degrees in a 9 x 3 inch
pan.

Yield: 12 servings

	RCU	FU	CAL	%F	P	F	C	NA
per serving	0	0	178	6	5	1	38	90

Bran Muffins - Kay Cavender

In a large bowl place:
2 C All Bran   2 C boiling water
1 quart buttermilk   1 1/2 C apple juice
3 eggs   2 1/2 C unsweetened
                                                    applesauce
3 tsp salt   4 tsp soda
4 C raisin bran   5 C whole wheat flour

Beat until mixture will thicken. Can be kept in refrigerator for 2 months. Bake at 350 degrees about 20 minutes.

Yield: 12 muffins

	RCU	FU	CAL	%F	P	F	C	NA
per muffin	0	0	80	7	3	1	15	112

Aunt Anne's Sugarless Cookies

With just a few changes from Aunt Anne's original recipe, this great tasting cookie will fool even your sugar lovers.

1 cup raisins
1 cup chopped apples

1/4 cup butter or margarine
1 tsp vanilla
1 tsp baking soda
1/2 cup chopped walnuts, optional

1/2 cup dates
1 cup frozen unsweetened
pear-apple or apple concentrate
2 large egg whites
2 cup whole wheat flour
1 cup rolled oats

Boil raisins, dates and apples in juice concentrate for 10 minutes. Add butter to hot mixture; let cool. Place fruit mixture in mixing bowl. Add egg whites and vanilla; beat well. Add flour, soda, and oats; beat well. Stir in nuts. Drop by teaspoonfuls onto cookie sheet that has been sprayed with vegetable coating. Bake in 350 degree oven for 12 minutes or until lightly golden brown on top.

Yield: 48 cookies

Note: This recipe was taken from the book "Desserts to Lower Your Fat Thermostat" with permission of the author, Barbara W. Higa. Published by Vitality House International, 1675 North Freedom Blvd. 11-C, Provo, Utah 84604. Paperback, $12.95.

	RCU	FU	CAL	%F	P	F	C	NA
per cookie	0	0	59	19	1	1	11	32

Decreasing the cost of Meals

Good wholesome eating can be relatively inexpensive if the amount of meat is decreased and a number of staple foods are added to the diet. Following are some general ideas to reduce food costs.

...Buy the staple items like rice, beans and wheat in bulk. Substantial savings can be made this way and you will also be dependent on the stores if an emergency arises.

...Eat more meals at home. Home-cooked meals are much cheaper than restaurant meals.

...Use meats less often and in smaller amounts. These are usually the most expensive food items.

...Buy extra food that you use when it comes on sale.

...Buy fewer convenience and snack foods. They are not usually appropriate anyway.

...Take lunches when convenient. You can be assured of getting good wholesome food that conforms to the guidelines.

...Grow a garden when possible. Even a small plot can grow a large number of vegetables which both taste better and save money.

...Preserve your own fruits. Commercially canned or frozen fruits usually have too much sugar. You can reduce the amount of sugar dramatically when you preserve your own.

Altering Recipes

Any recipe can be altered to better conform to good management principles. As your taste for salt and sweets changes, you will find it preferable to change for taste as well as for thinness and health. Sugars can be eliminated or greatly reduced. Honey can be substituted for sugar (since half the honey will give the same sweetness as sugar). In a recipe, you can use one-fourth the amount of honey, or even less if you choose. Honey can change the taste and texture, so experiment a bit to determine how much to use. Frozen fruit juice or fructose can be used in place of sugar, providing fewer calories, yet providing sweetness.

Whole wheat flour can be substituted for white flour. In bread or other items where this flour is the major item, some difference in technique may be required. In making bread, the dough needs to be kneaded or mixed longer to develop the gluten so that it will hold together.

Yogurt or blended cottage cheese can replace some cream in vegetable dishes or salad dressings. Buttermilk or skim milk can be used instead of whole milk. Low-fat mayonnaise or light margarine can be used to save fat calories. The amount of oil in recipes can be decreased. You can use fat-free chicken stock (cooled and skimmed) to replace oil or butter in cooking.

Your own imagination is the only limiting factor in how many improvements can be made. Most of the recipes in this section have been altered from existing recipes.

Appendix Ten
Model of WRM

All scientists feel a necessity to develop a "model" that explains how a new idea works. The purpose of this appendix is to present our model for those of you who are more scientifically oriented.

Many of the ideas relating to this model have been discussed in other parts of the book and will not be reintroduced here. However, we will try to pull the ideas together so that you can better understand the functioning of this critical system.

Figure A10.1 shows our concept of the model. Note that body weight is controlled by the weight regulating mechanism (WRM) through increasing or decreasing the appetite and by wasting or conserving energy (boxes below the dashed line). How the body regulates eating is discussed in Appendix 2 and the energy wasting and conserving mechanisms are explained in Appendix 3.

Figure A10.1

Weight Regulating Mechanism

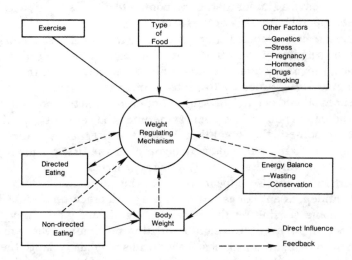

These are powerful regulators that are used by the WRM to resist a change in body weight at all costs. If the setpoint goes up or down, the WRM signals these two boxes to make whatever change necessary to cause the weight to go down or up to match the setpoint. If the setpoint is simply too high (as in obesity) normal dietary techniques will cause a decrease in the fat stores which will cause the WRM to increase the drive to eat and slow down energy use to help maintain setpoint weight.

The boxes above the dotted line are factors that can affect the setpoint of the WRM. The most important of these factors in terms of weight control is exercise. The body probably interprets inactivity as a threat to survivability and increases the setpoint so the system can store fat. It also changes the metabolism and makes other changes to protect the fat until the organism gets active again. The role of inactivity in setting the WRM is discussed in some detail in Appendix 4, Factors Contributing to Obesity and in Chapter Two. Chapter Two also discusses the value of exercise in weight control in addition to decreasing the setpoint.

The second most important factor in resetting the WRM is shown in the box labeled "Type of Food." There is no doubt about the role of rich foods, fats, and refined carbohydrates in resetting the WRM. Rats fed the so-called "supermarket diet" gain excess weight rapidly. Most of us have a similar diet. For a complete discussion of food factors see Appendix 3 and Chapter Three.

The last box is labeled simply "Other Factors." These factors do affect the setpoint of the WRM, but many cannot be controlled. For instance, pregnancy almost always adjusts the setpoint of the WRM to a higher level, probably to protect both the baby and mother if hard times should occur. The setpoint often returns to a normal level after the baby is born. However, sometimes the setpoint appears to "stick" at some higher level than before the pregnancy and resists coming back to normal. This may occur after the first pregnancy or may not occur until after several babies are carried.

Certain drugs also appear to adjust the setpoint. For instance, some antidepressant drugs have a strong influence on weight and many people starting on them make a significant gain. They probably act directly on the weight-regulating mechanism through the action of some neurohormones. These drugs may also change the activity level since they are rather sedating. Amphetamines and some of the other appetite-suppressant drugs may actually lower the setpoint of the WRM since studies show little difference in food intake as a result of taking the drugs. People taking appetite suppressants tend to decrease their weight by 10 to 20 pounds while on the drugs, but return quickly to their old weight when the medication is stopped. A two-year study using appetite suppressants showed a quick loss of 15 pounds or so on the average, followed by a two-year period of stable weight at the lower level. As soon as the medication was stopped, the weight quickly returned to and stabilized at the former level. The problem is that the long-term use of these medications is almost certain to cause addiction in a high percentage of users. The withdrawal may be associated with severe depression and suicidal tendencies.

All appetite suppressants are approved by the FDA for short-term use only, i.e., a few weeks, and thus clinical use for a longer period is not approved. A physician may be guilty of malpractice by continuing to use medication for a prolonged period when it is not approved for that usage. We feel that the risks of the medication far outweigh any benefit obtained by stabilizing at a lighter weight, especially when the setpoint of the WRM can more effectively be lowered by exercise and changes in food selection.

It has been known for years that people who stop smoking usually gain weight. The theory has been that more food is eaten because it tastes better or that food is used for oral gratification instead of cigarettes. Although these factors may contribute, there is evidence that the setpoint may be lowered by smoking, and often seems to be raised to a higher level when smoking stops.

Before anyone gets the idea that smoking is a useful tool to control weight, we hasten to point out the following factors: The health risks of smoking far outweigh the risks of being heavy. If you want to smoke to look better by being thinner, the premature aging of the skin associated with smoking may make you look a lot older and make you look a lot worse than if you were slightly heavier with nice skin. Exercise will do a much better job of lowering the WRM and has healthy side effects instead of negative ones. If you think that smoking and exercise together might be useful, you should know that smoking will reduce both the inclination and the ability to exercise effectively. Exercising and smoking together are not likely to be as effective as exercising alone. We have seen many smokers who gained weight after stopping, went back to smoking to lose weight, but found that the smoking didn't really help.

Even dieting can affect the setpoint and is frequently followed by a gain in weight to a level higher than before. As mentioned earlier, a decrease in food intake below that needed to maintain the body weight at setpoint results in an increased appetite and a decrease in energy wasting. Of course, if a person is really starving, this mechanism is truly important, allowing the person to adapt to the next episode of starvation by having an even larger amount of fat stores, as well as having a body designed to protect those fat stores. The problem is, the WRM can't distinguish between starvation and dieting. These adaptive responses that protected our ancestors from periods of starvation may lie dormant for long periods and cause no particular problem until triggered by a period of unwise dietary efforts. It may be that dieting is more responsible for producing obesity than overeating. An example of how this can happen may be helpful. If a person who has a stable body weight is eating roughly 2,000 calories a day and decides to lose weight, he may go to 1,500 calories. The weight-regulating mechanism recognizes that the food intake has decreased and that the body weight is starting to fall. In an attempt to defend the weight, the body starts conserving energy and stimulates the appetite. The weight loss soon stops even if the dieter can resist the stronger urges to eat. If the person gives up and goes back to his original 2,000 calories, the body weight may increase because it now uses less energy. If the dieter wants to continue losing, he must further reduce his food intake, perhaps to 1,000 or 1,200 calories. Even then, weight loss will eventually stop. When the eating returns to even 1,500 calories, the weight will perhaps increase again to its previous normal level, since the body has become so much more efficient. Of course, the problem is compounded if the stress of dieting moves the setpoint to a higher level as well.

Emotional stress, certain hormones and even a mineral deficiency can affect the setpoint of the WRM. These three factors are covered in Appendix 4.

It is obvious from this discussion that the control of body weight is a complex and well-controlled response. Luckily, the setpoint can be lowered by conscious effort on your part and persistent weight changes can be made.

Appendix Eleven
Old Ideas vs. New

If you are a seasoned dieter, you will notice many differences between old traditional ideas and the new concepts. To be successful in reprogramming your body, you really do need to make some changes in your thinking and in your attitude.

Following are a few very common ideas and attitudes about dieting and weight loss together with the way in which we would like you to look at the same issues.

Old Idea: If you are fat, you have been overeating or are too lazy. You don't have enough willpower and have not been trying hard enough or you would be thin.

New Concept: These ideas only result in guilt and faulty dietary practices. Obesity is seldom due simply to overeating. Even prolonged force-feeding only produces a few pounds of fat gain and usually does not lead to obesity. Although most obese people eat out of control at times, this is a natural response to periods of food restriction. Obesity occurs when your body is programmed to be fat with a high setpoint and many defenses against starvation which conserve energy and protect fat stores. "Laziness" is usually a result of your body conserving energy and not being able or willing to produce enough energy for you to be very active. Few people can win out over these powerful controls that tend to keep the fat levels too high. Most restrictive diets and attempts to control weight only result in more fatness. Large amounts of excess fat usually don't occur without many attempts to diet or without eating irregular meals. We now view grossly obese people as people who have tried very hard to lose weight, and feel that most of them would only be slightly overweight if they had never tried to diet.

Old Idea: To lose weight, you must cut down your caloric intake. The more you cut back, the faster you will lose fat and the better you will do. Missing meals entirely saves calories and helps you to lose fat more quickly.

New Concept: Both eating too few calories and going long periods without eating seem to trigger your body's defenses against starvation. In the long term, this only raises the setpoint, makes your body conserve energy more effectively and makes you fatter.

Old Idea: Calories are all equal. A piece of cake will affect you just the same as 375 calories of salad or other food. Save your calories for something that you really would enjoy.

New Concept: The quality of the food in the long term is more important than the caloric value. High sugar and fat diets seem to raise the setpoint and both are effectively converted to body fat. Sugar causes insulin excess and short satiety period, leading to hunger shortly after eating.

Old Idea: An effective reducing diet must involve an exact number of calories, a menu plan which must be followed precisely, and a list of forbidden foods. Whenever you eat a few extra calories, eat differently from the planned menu, or eat a forbidden food, you are "cheating." If you "cheat" even a little, you have "screwed up" the entire day. You might as well really eat and enjoy it since you have already "blown it." You can start again tomorrow.

Truth: Artificial guidelines for the calorie amount and exact foods to be eaten are difficult to follow and usually don't produce desired results. It seems best not to think of foods as being absolutely forbidden. Attaching moral values to eating only produces guilt and poor self-esteem. Modify only those foods and eating patterns that are a problem, and choose your own foods—foods that you can enjoy and live with for a lifetime. An occasional indiscretion with foods makes little difference in the long run. As you get into harmony with your eating drives, cravings and binge eating will not be a problem. You should never think of being on or off a diet.

Old Idea: You must live with hunger to be successful. Being hungry indicates that you are doing well and losing fat. Eating means giving in and not having enough willpower.

New Concept: Prolonged hunger merely triggers starvation defenses and leads to binge eating. Eating is essential and should be enjoyed whenever there is a need for food (which may be every few hours). A normal relationship with food will produce much better long-term results.

Old Idea: If you have eaten within the last four to six hours, any desire to eat couldn't possibly by physical and must therefore be psychological.

New Concept: There are many conditions in which true physical hunger can be present very shortly after eating. Understanding the functioning of your body will allow you to better identify true hunger.

Old Idea: It is best to ignore hunger. Find ways to keep busy and keep your mind off your hunger. Don't give in to it. You will then be able to eat less and lose weight.

New Concept: Ignoring hunger only stimulates starvation defenses and often leads to binge eating. You should really pay attention to your hunger and eat as needed to supply your body with the energy and nutrients that it "requests" of you.

Old Idea: Exercise helps only by burning calories. You burn only 300 calories by walking for an hour. It is much easier to cut back that many calories instead. That will balance out the energy equation and the end result will be the same.

New Concept: Calorie burning is way down the list of important functions for exercise. Exercise produces many profound changes and is essential to effective weight control. Cutting back calories even with exercise creates many problems and prevents the desired changes.

Appendix Twelve
How Psychological Factors Affect Weight

Throughout this book, obesity has been discussed as a physiological condition. Psychological factors such as low self-esteem, anger, depression, guilt, boredom, and loneliness can also contribute to obesity. Various psychological conflicts are also factors in the obese process. These psychological factors influence obesity in the following ways.

Psychological problems can lead to overeating. By itself, this overeating should only lead to a modest weight gain. Many thin people overeat in response to psychological factors and don't gain weight. Large weight gain probably only occurs with alternating overeating with dietary efforts so that the setpoint is frequently adjusted higher to compensate for episodes of perceived starvation.

Psychological problems and conflict are a form of stress. Stress can move the setpoint higher. Many of our patients have reported sudden unexplained weight gains after various types of psycholgical stress such as following the death of a loved one, a divorce, a move, an episode of depression, or similar disturbing situation. In many cases, patients are adamant that no change in eating patterns have occurred, and often gain occurs in spite of less eating.

Stress induced by psychological conflict makes hormonal and other biochemical changes. Stress hormones including adrenalin, noradrenalin, and cortisol increase insulin resistance. These maladaptive changes that lead to increased fat stores may occur as a protective mechanism in response to various types of situations perceived by the weight-regulating mechanism as threatening.

Psychological factors often lead to decreased activity, which has a well-known effect in raising the setpoint. Psychic conflict produces an energy "drain" which leaves little energy or desire for exercise. Psychological problems may disorganize your life and make it difficult to schedule regular exercise periods. Trying to solve these psychological problems may take priority over exercise.

Psychological blockers may interfere with following an effective weight-management program. If weight loss is considered threatening by your subconscious mind, it will attempt to stop you from succeeding by encouraging you to eat inappropriately. The conflict between conscious wishes to stay on a program to become thin and the subconscious effort to keep you fat may cause a lot of stress which in turn contributes to obesity.

Many of the psychological problems that are often associated with obesity seem to be caused by the obese process, dietary efforts to lose the weight, or by repeated failure to lose weight permanently. Some psychological factors that contribute to obesity will be discussed.

Low Self-esteem

Low self-esteem is one of the most common and possibly the most debilitating of all the mental states associated with being overweight. Research suggests that the fatter you are, the lower will be your self-esteem. Self-esteem consists of the accumulation of "self-statements" you have made about yourself over a lifetime. These self-statements reflect what parents, siblings, teachers, employers, peers, and others have said about you. They also reflect self-judgments regarding body image, talents, and worthiness. Self-esteem, therefore, reflects how you feel that you measure up to some real or imagined standard. It is not uncommon to find yourself very exacting in certain areas of life if you are overweight. Your standards for comparison may be very rigorous and feelings of worthlessness often follow overeating. The more your body differs from your ideal, the more worthless you feel. You may be very successful in your vocation, in raising a family or following some other pursuit, but these successes often seem insignifiant in view of your failure to achieve a certain body build. It is not unusual for a normal weight young girl who has a healthy body and who is eating according to the indications of her weight-regulating mechanism to be told that she needs to lose five or ten pounds in order to make the drill team. Although there is no good physiological basis for the drill team's weight goal, it may instill a feeling of inadequacy and later a lowering of self-esteem in the girl.

One approach to this problem is that if you feel inferior to those around you or if you never quite measure up to your own personal standard of thinness, examine the standard. Rather than assuming that you should weight a certain weight, determine your weight according to your own lean body mass rather than some outdated height-weight table or other standard.

Another result of low self-esteem can be eating as a reaction to criticism. One way of dealing with criticism is to dispute in your own mind what is said. If a professor tells you that you have failed a test, you cannot translate this into proof that you are stupid. Rather than accepting the grade as proof that you are dumb, you might say something like, "This is not proof of my lack of intelligence and only represents a small sample of my understanding." You need to appreciate your good qualities and seek out people who give you positive feedback. As you accept yourself and feed your self-esteem with credit for work well done, you will find yourself free to work on new accomplishments, among which will be a thinner body.

Anger

Anger is an interesting emotion and one that can prove very counterproductive in terms of controlling weight. Anger not only appears to have a psychological tendency to make you overeat but may have a physiological effect leading to low blood sugar and subsequent overeating from this effect. Adrenalin is produced as you become angry and your blood sugar level increases as you prepare to fight or to run away. Adrenalin prevents insulin from being produced but as soon as the anger passes, the adrenalin quickly leaves the system, insulin production rapidly increases, and the excess blood sugar is converted to body fat. Although you may not eat while aroused by anger, you may eat too much after the anger has been replaced by neutral feelings.

One of the best ways to cope with anger is to exercise. If you find yourself angry, take a brisk walk, chop wood, or play a hard game of racquetball. An even better approach is to avoid anger. Since it is your mind that makes you angry and not the activating event itself, you can choose to either be angry or not. Another way to avoid anger is to avoid dieting. Research has shown a significant relationship between anger and percent body fat in people when dieting regularly. Obviously, anger in any form will be detrimental to your efforts to control weight.

Depression

Depression has been described as anger turned inward. It may have many of the same components as anger only instead of being directed toward someone else, it is directed toward yourself. It is normal for your emotions to fluctuate from day to day. It is not unusual to be on top of the world one day and feeling blue the next. Depression in the overweight person may be a pervasive feeling of gloom and worthlessness. Fatigue and lassitude may make each day appear insurmountable. Food may make you feel a little better, so continuous eating becomes mandatory in order to simply survive another day. As diets are begun and quickly abandoned, you feel more of a failure and more worthless. Depression becomes incapacitating, and you neglect proper care of your home, children and yourself.

Serious depression should never be lightly dismissed. It is our suggestion that if you are seriously depressed, you seek proper medical attention. As the depression clears up, it will be easier for you to cope with life without having to overuse food. For those who are depressed but still functioning more or less in a normal manner, we suggest that the walking, jogging, or other exercise programs previously outlined will be very beneficial. Walking is something almost everyone can do and should help lift your spirits. As you walk regularly, your energy level will improve and the depression will be reduced.

Proper self-talk will also prove beneficial. Self-talk in depressed, overweight people focuses on what a mess they have made of their lives, how hopeless everything is, and how impossible it is to change. It is possible to dispute these self-statements. Examine the standards by which you are measuring yourself. They are probably based upon false ideas. Refuse to think these false ideas. Build a high wall around your self-esteem and don't let any ''garbage'' ideas over the wall into your garden of self-esteem. As you allow your self-esteem to grow, give yourself credit for being a worthwhile individual. It is hard for you to be angry at someone you feel is worthwhile and for whom you have tremendous respect. This increased self-esteem should help improve your depression. Refuse to accept all the ''shoulds'' that have been running (and ruining) your life up to now. Take a fresh look at these imperatives and remake them so that they reflect a fair and attainable standard by which you may honestly evaluate your behavior. As you begin to accept and love yourself, you will find that others will react toward you in a better fashion. Accept the compliments and kindnesses of others. You will find the depression melting away and your energy level improving. As this process occurs, you will be more able to control problem eating.

Guilt

Guilt may be classified as a symptom stress or a negative feeling resulting from judgments you make on your own acts. In this case, your own improper eating is not acceptable as something that normally occurs. Instead, you castigate yourself and end up feeling guilt or shame. Guilt is so uncomfortable that you eventually feel you must have relief and resort to the short-term relief of eating. A destructive cycle is therefore initiated. The concept of a weight-regulating mechanism is very helpful in dealing with guilt. By accepting the fact that your eating is largely governed by internal neural and chemical mechanisms, you do not have to feel guilty for eating. By accepting that the eating was requested by the weight-regulating mechanism, guilt is removed and you are spared subsequent eating bouts.

Boredom

It is not uncommon to encounter people who report eating out of simple boredom. For these people, food becomes a form of entertainment. Boredom may be a rather complex mental or emotional state. It often occurs in people of above average intelligence who may not be satisfied with the visual or auditory messages normal to everyday life but seek the sensations of different temperatures, tastes, smells, and feelings that food can provide. Many of these people do not realize that it is not hunger that is leading them to eat excessively but a form of boredom.

One patient bought an indoor exercise bike that he rode in the evening whenever he felt bored. His problem eating almost disappeared and he lowered his setpoint as he improved his fitness level. You may experience boredom when you feel that what you are doing is uninteresting or dull. Many young people are easily bored and are unable to bear the passage of time without TV, loud music or some other form of entertainment. On the other hand, many adults feel bored by television and other "canned" forms of stimulation. Some people seem to thrive on repetition and can find challenge in doing simple things over and over. You may gain insight into your emotions of boredom by looking at your ability to anticipate the finished product. Some people have a problem delaying gratification and must have the reinforcement immediately. Others seem to be able to see the finished product from its various stages of completion.

Handwork is a good example. If each stitch were viewed as the total product, it is not likely that anyone would ever knit a sweater. By visualizing each stitch as bringing you closer to the beautiful sweater, you remain interested in your work and find great satisfaction as the task is finished.

Others who are bored easily may be telling themselves something like: "I can't stand doing the same thing over and over" or "I'll go crazy if I have to read another word." By becoming aware of what you are saying to yourself, you may be able to dispute what you are programming into your subconcious. Try saying something like, "I prefer doing a variety of things but I can stand this repetition because it brings me closer to my goal." By breaking down tasks into smaller units, you may be able to find satisfaction as each unit is accomplished and thereby reduce boredom.

Loneliness

Most people experience loneliness at some time or another in their lives. This feeling may be very unpleasant and leads them to almost any length to avoid feeling lonely. They may join bowling leagues, take ceramic classes, go to singles bars, or remarry the same person for the third time all in the hope of filling the void that being alone creates. Others use eating to help them escape. Overeating may lead to shame and guilt which compounds the problem. Loneliness may also be accompanied by depression which makes it difficult to do anything positive about weight control. If life is hopeless, why struggle with dieting? Overeating in this situation may also trigger shame and guilt which makes it that much harder to deal with the loneliness. You may feel so negative toward yourself that other people seem to go out of their way to avoid you. Often, the more you need companionship, the more you seem to put barriers between yourself and others.

While some relief from loneliness may be found from seeking more social interactions with peers from work, church, or a club, it is unlikely that these social interactions will remove the emptiness experienced when you are at home alone. Many people have found a pet to be a nondemanding companion that can occupy the empty hours in exchange for a minimum amount of care. For some, a cat or a small dog that can be kept indoors may be very helpful. Others might like a larger dog which could accompany them on their walks or other physical activities. Such animals are intelligent but never nag or mistreat you.

Some people may simply need to readjust their mental programming. Many people live very satifying lives by themselves. They can be fascinating people who have many friends and are interested in other people. They may be widows who accept their new marital status as being completely natural. They do not feel worthless simply because they are alone. Many are active in volunteer organizations, civic groups, or church groups. They have friends who visit or call occasionally. They often seem busy and hardly have time to take care of their own necessities. Because they are interesting to others,they are not lonely but find themselves occupied by interesting thoughts and activities. Eating may be done at home or outside the home but rarely out of boredom or loneliness.

This suggests that living alone doesn't have to be seen as a horrible prison sentence. If you look at your self-talk, it is likely that you are saying something like, "It is awful being alone all the time and I can't stand it. I have to get away from this terrible feeling." You can dispute these ideas with something like, "I prefer having fun companions with whom to share my life. However, rather than feeling sorry for myself, I will work on making myself the most attractive and interesting person I can be. This will maximize my chances of finding an acceptable companion but, more importantly, will help me to be better company when I am alone." By actively disputing the desire to eat undue amounts of food simply because you are alone, you will increase your ability to be in harmony with the drives from the weight-regulating mechanism and obtain an ideal body weight.

The dynamics of eating due to these mental states are made much worse if you constantly eat below the drives of your weight-regulating mechanism. These emotional states interfere with your ability to resist food and often encourage you to "binge eat" once you have eaten some forbidden goodie. On the other hand, these emotions are much less of a problem if you are eating enough to satisfy the eating drives of your weight-regulating mechanism.

Psychological Blockers

In addition to these five emotional states which are often assocated with nondirected eating there are certain mental states which may prevent a person from following any program that will result in successful weight loss. We refer to these subconcious states as psychological blockers. These blockers are activated in some people when they contemplate or begin a change in behavior that would result in weight loss and manifest themselves as extreme anxiety. These people become frustrated because the only way they know to relieve the anxiety is to overeat. The psychological blockers may be classified into four types: power, punishing, sex, and miscellaneous. If you have experienced a powerful anxiety attack when dieting and have been unable to stay on a reasonable diet for any length of time, it is possible that a psychological block is in place. You are advised to consult a professional who has had experience in helping others overcome this type of problem.

Power

Fatness may often be an issue in a power struggle between a child and a parent or between marriage partners. A child may find that being fat is something that upsets his parents who otherwise are able to exert powerful control over him. It is a way of sabotaging the parental directives without being obviously rebellious. Unfortunately, the anxiety related to eating small quantities of food continues long after the child is grown and is no longer under the dominant influence of the parents. It is not uncommon to encounter a person who was relatively thin until a certain age, who then rapidly gained over 50 pounds and who has since been unable to return to a normal weight.

Alice reported being normal weight until the seventh grade. Between the seventh and eighth grades she gained 100 pounds. She detests her father and finds it very hard to be around him. There are periods of her life immediately preceding her weight gain that she cannot recall. Although it is possible that a sex-related blocker is operating here, it was determined that a power blocker developed in an effort to subvert the dominant and controlling nature of her father. Even though Alice no longer lives at home, she has not been able to get her weight below 220 pounds. A loss of a few pounds is enough to start a binge which more than restores the lost weight. As therapy proceeded, Alice found a reason to discontinue treatment as the focus on the core problem became very uncomfortable for her. It is unlikely that Alice will ever be able to reach her ideal weight until this power-related psychological blocker is resolved through professional aid.

Sometimes the psychological blockers operate in the spouse and not in the patient. We often see women whose husbands sabotage their dieting efforts. Whenever their wives go on a diet, these men bring home candy and other tasty foods. They tempt them with favorite dishes while watching TV or invite them to restaurants where large, high-calorie meals are served. In some cases, eating together is the only common bond in a realtionship and the husband is very deliberate in doing things to keep his wife fat. At other times, these acts are done subconciously. The psychological blockers for these men may involve a preference for larger women or a fear of losing her should she become more attractive. Unhappily, the strength of the blockers in the spouse is often so great that few people are able to lose their weight without major changes in the relationship. Some are able to achieve a healthier relationship and maintain ideal weight. Most, however, continue to suffer from low self-esteem, depression and overweight because of their dependency upon the spouse who is unwilling or unable to make any adjustments in his own life. If you are encountering a sabotage-type blocker in your spouse, you will need a very supportive counselor as you start on your goal of obtaining ideal weight. It probably would be helpful to have your spouse involved in the process with you.

Punishment

Although not as common as power or sex-related blockers, punishment-related blockers do occur. If a punishing psychological blocker is active in your eating pattern, you will probably hate your body and feel it is something horrible that needs to be degraded. Sometimes when you are binging, you may experience a separation of your body from yourself. It will seem that the body has its own volition and is eating without any effort on your part. As you eat, you feel more ugly and despise yourself more and more.

Almost no one consciously chooses to become fat, but the subconcious may drive you to it for various reasons. Perhaps the subconscious perceives you as sinful or bad because of some unacceptable behavior. Becoming fat may be the form of punishment chosen to make up for your sins. You may be conscious of the unhappiness your overweight state causes and try hard to control it, but, failing to understand the needs of the subconscious, you decide that you have no willpower and are doomed to being fat forever. The very contest between your conscious and subconscious may produce the unhappiness that satisfies your need to be punished. Hence, you make use of dieting as the arena in which to act out your conflict. A concerned mother in describing her unhappy 14-year-old son's eating behavior suggested that it appeared he was trying to kill himself with food. At 335 pounds, he may well be succeeding if this is his subconscious drive.

A wife whose husband wants her thin and sexy may purposely choose to become fat as a form of punishment to her husband. He may tend to see her as a possession more than as a person. She may feel that he doesn't appreciate her, abuses her, and treats her unfairly. He may be staying out late with the boys and spending a disproportionate share of the money. Becoming fat is one of the few things she can do to hurt or punish him. As a man with a fat wife, he is deprived of any social prestige he might have gained if she were more attractive. The wife's needs to be thin are thus outweighed by her need to get back at her husband. Before this woman can lose her weight she and her husband will need help from a professional to resolve the hidden agendas of their relationship.

Sex

The professional literature reports many cases in which sex-related psychological blockers actively prevented women from losing weight. Many women hold the misconception that fat is an effective defense from a male's sexual advances. They seem to think that if they are fat, they will be ugly enough that no man would be interested in them. In these cases, the woman is often able to begin a successful diet and lose weight rather easily until her feminine curves appear. At that point, she experiences significant anxiety and finds herself binging on highly fattening foods. The diet is abandoned and fat is soon higher than ever.

Mary, a 19-year-old girl, spent most of the summer at a "fat camp" in a mountain resort and lost considerable weight. While taking a walk, she ran into a boy from her former high school. Although they had never gone together, she had been and was still attracted to this young man. Even though no advances were made, she felt uneasy and threatened. As soon as they parted company, she bought a large amount of candy and began eating as much as possible. Subconsiously, and perhaps even consciously, she felt threatened by the thought of forming a relationship with a man. Somehow, the encounter threatened her psychologically secure position and set in motion strong drives to abandon dieting and return to her normal, fat condition.

Another rather naive patient was quite overweight when she married in her mid-twenties. When normal marital relations were not established, her husband explained that he would care for and provide for her, but that there was no way that anyone could make love to someone with such a grotesque body. After a quick annulment, she felt a strong need to prove to herself that she was sexually acceptable. She abandoned her previous moral standards and proved through a number of promiscuous relationships that there were indeed men to whom she was sexually aceptable.

However, one cannot easily dismiss a lifetime of moral teachings and her subconscious did not accept her promiscuity. Within a short time, she had put on an extra 100 pounds of fat. This may have been the result of her subconscious desperately driving her to put on enough weight to make her unattractive to men and therefore stop her unacceptable behaviors. These two examples of sex-related psychological blockers may help you understand the complex and often subconcscious nature of these conditions and realize the importance of consulting a qualified professional for help in dealing with them.

Miscellaneous

Other forms of psychological blockers exist and we will describe a few we have encountered. A child or a spouse may do almost anything, including becoming fat, to get attention. Even severe punishment or constant nagging are better than being ignored. Norma was a teenager from a large family whose busy mother was perplexed when Norma began to gain weight. Her mother had always had high expectations for Norma and she began taking her to every weight-control program imaginable. She would fix special meals, watch her closely and even do a lot of exercise with Norma, all to no avail. Norma didn't lose any weight even though she claimed to be eating only 500 to 600 calories per day. A test at a local university revealed that she had a normal metabolic rate. She admitted deceiving everyone to get attention from her mother who otherwise might not have taken time from her busy schedule to spend with Norma.

Food may represent security to you. One patient described how many of her happy childhood memories involved food. She remembered sitting around a fire with her family eating treats. On weekends they would drive into town as a family for something to eat. Holidays involved going to her grandparents for big holiday dinners. Suddenly, everything changed. Her older brothers and sisters all moved away, her parents divorced and her mother became an invalid. She was left alone at age 9 or 10 to prepare her own meals. The only part of her happy childhood she could recapture was the eating part. She attempted to make herself happy by treating herself with food. She used eating to relieve the emptiness and bordom she now felt. Every time she tried to diet, she felt lonely, deprived and very unhappy.

Some overweight people have a real fear of becoming thin. They are afraid that more will be expected of them and that they will be forced into competing with others who are more competent. They may have a fear that even if they were thin, that they would still be unacceptable to others. It may seem that being fat is safer and less likely to get them into uncomfortable, competitive situtations. This and many other mental states can prevent a person from succeeding in attaining a more ideal weight.

A technique that has been helpful to many patients with this and similar conditions is listening to their own self-talk. If you listen closely to the line of reasoning you are using, you may get an understanding of what is operating in your subconscious. You may be saying things that give you permission to eat. A classic example is, "Well, I've already blown it today. I may as well enjoy myself and try again tomorrow." Something that may not be verbalized, even internally, may be a thought such as, "It is not fair that everyone gets to eat all the birthday cake they want and I can only drink this nasty water." Such thoughts make you feel more and more deprived and mistreated. It usually doesn't take you long to make a logical reason why you should go ahead and eat some of that cake and ice cream. By carefully trying to tell yourself out loud what you are saying inside you may see that the self-talk is illogical. Using logic, you can dispute the reasoning and enable yourself to eat more rationally.

Dealing With Psychological Problems

It is beyond the scope of this book to deal extensively with psychological problems. Some suggestions have been given about dealing with minor problems. Major problems should really be dealt with through appropriate professional counselors. The continued stress of unresolved psychological conflict will probably interfere with your attempt to lower your weight setpoint.

Behavior Modification

Behavior modification has become the cornerstone of obesity management for over 15 years and is often used in conjunction with various diet plans. In view of new understanding about obesity management, the whole concept of behavior modification needs to be reevaluated and updated. Albert J. Stunkard, a well-known authority on weight control has made the following statements about behavior modification:

"Behavioral therapy has not fully realized the bright hopes that were held out for it in the early days. A common response to such disappointment is to return to the basics and to review the assumptions on which the treatment was based. Precisely this course has been taken by two leading theorists in recent reviews of the status of the behavioral treatment of obesity (Mahoney, 1978; Wilson, 1980). Each found that many, if not most, of the assumptions (both explicit and implicit) on which the behavioral treatment of obesity was based were invalid. Mahoney has summarized six such assumptions (1978):

1. Obesity is a learning disorder, created by and amenable to principles of conditioning.
2. Obesity is a simple disorder resulting from excess caloric intake.
3. The obese individual is an overeater.
4. Obese persons are more sensitive to food stimuli than are nonobese individuals.
5. There are important differences in the "eating style" of obese and nonobese persons.
6. Training an obese person to behave like a nonobese one will result in weight loss."

(International Handbook of Behavior Modification and Therapy, Bellacle, Hersen and Kozden, 1982, pg. 657.)

In addition to the flawed major assumptions upon which behavior modification principles are based, many mistaken minor concepts have been used in formulating treatment principles. Although behavior modification does produce modest success, the observed weight loss does not seem to result from the suggested behavioral changes.

Some very brilliant and creative minds formulated behavior modification principles using the state-of-the-art concepts of 15 years ago. A similar creative effort using current understanding of obesity may provide a great deal of help for implementing the general treatment principles outlined in this book.

Appendix Thirteen
Table of Food Composition

Reprograming Plan — Summary

1) Exercise will lower the setpoint. It will also increase the muscle mass, increase the metabolic rate, increase the fat-burning enzymes, decrease insulin resistence, decrease appetite, and increase energy level. These bodily changes are best seen in long distance runners who often get their body fat to very low levels. Although we are not sure exactly what causes this long distance running effect, other similar activities seem to produce the same changes. Alternative activities must use large muscles groups, be steady and rhythmic, keep the heart rate between 70 and 80 percent of maximum, be prolonged for 30 to 60 minutes and be done often, preferably daily. Walking, jogging, running, cycling, swimming, aerobic dancing, skipping, and some exercise machines (such as mini-trampolines, treadmills, rowing machines, or exercise cycles) all can be effective.

2) Decrease the fat in your diet. Excess dietary fats are now known to be major causes of diseases such as certain cancers, arteriosclerosis, and diabetes. High fat intake raises the setpoint, and a low-fat diet will lower the setpoint. The average American diet contains about 40 to 50 percent fat, which is two to four times higher than the ideal. Ten to 20 percent fat is recommended. There are a number of ways of reducing fats: Reduce fats by decreasing butter, oil, salad dressings, fried foods, and meats, etc. as much as possible. The column in the main text entitled "% Ft" will indicate the high-fat foods. Anything with higher fat content than 20 percent may need to be eaten with lower fat foods or in smaller quantities.

3) Decrease your intake of refined carbohydrates. This will lower the setpoint and help to control insulin levels. Artificial sweeteners and caffeine should also be avoided. The point system will help you recognize foods containing refined carbohydrates. Reading labels on prepared foods should point out hidden sugars.

4) Reduce intake of high calorie-density foods. These foods have a lot of calories packed into a small volume. By the time you have eaten enough high calorie-dense foods to satisfy your need for chewing and tasting and stomach filling, you may have ingested excessive calories which can produce body fat. Fats have nine calories per gram (compared to the four calories per gram for carbohydrate and protein). This makes them very calorically dense. Most fats contain little water which increases caloric density even higher. Sugar has been dehydrated and stripped of fiber making it calorically dense. Various dehydrated foods (like dried fruit and beef jerky) or foods naturally low in water content like nuts have high caloric density and need to be eaten in limited quantities. The column in the food description called RCal refers to relative calories, and gives the number of calories per 100 grams of each food item. This gives an excellent comparison between various foods and provides a good indication of caloric density.

5) Stop Faulty Drinking. Drinking calorie-containing fluids or eating in response to thirst often causes more energy intake than the body can waste leaving it no choice but to store the extra energy as fat. Most drinks are refined or processed so as to provide little chewing or satisfaction, and are consumed and absored quickly leading to insulin excess and a short satiety period. Drink water in response to thirst, eat solid food in response to hunger. Drinks high in caffeine turn sugars to body fat and should also be avoided.

6) Eat in harmony with the hunger drives of the body. Many people learn to use food for many reasons besides their biologic need for energy. Food can be used for comfort, companionship, pleasure, relaxation, relief of boredom, or for many other reasons. This type of eating may lead to fat gain and needs to be stopped.

It is also very important not to eat too little. If you consistently miss meals or eat less food than your body needs, various sensors throughout the body indicate to the weight-regulating mechanism that starvation conditions exist. A number of changes occur within the body to conserve energy and protect fat. These changes together with a possible raised setpoint may actually make your body fatter in the long term instead of reprograming it to be thinner.

Using Composition of Food Guideline

The Composition of Food table will be extremely useful in choosing and understanding healthy foods. This section should help you understand how to use the Table. The headings are explained below:

Item - Identifies the food item and the form in which it is described.

Portion - Amount or size of the food items listed. Sometimes expressed as a volume, sometimes as a weight, and sometimes a portion size.

RCU - Refined carbohydrate unit (explained in the Point System in chapter 4).

FU - Fat unit (explained in the Point System in chapter 4).

Cal - Calories (kilocalories) contained in the food.

RCal - Relative calories - number of calories per 100 grams.

This gives you an opportunity to compare foods which tend to come in different-sized portions on an equal basis (calories per 100 grams) and expresses the relative caloric density of each food item. Food with a low number (calorie per gram) tends to have a high water content and low fat content. The higher numbered foods are either high in fat, high in added sugars, low in water, or a combination of the above. It should be apparent which factor is the problem by looking at the "%Ft" column. For example, apricots have 51 calories per 100 grams when fresh, but increase to 260 calories per 100 grams when dried. Cooking techniques can be evaluated by comparing relative calories. Boiled potatoes have 80 calories per 100 grams. Baked potatoes lose a little water and become more calorically dense at 90 calories per 100 grams. Because of added fats, french fried potatoes have 274 calories per 100 grams. Potato chips which are dehydrated as well as having added fats are even worse at 568 calories per 100 grams.
The effect of adding sugar can also be seen. Fresh strawberries

have 37 calories per 100 grams. Frozen strawberries have added sugar and increase to 109 calories per 100 grams.

Snacks can also be compared in terms of caloric density. Peaches are 38 calories per 100 grams while peanuts have 585 calories per 100 grams-15 times as high. Keep in mind that the lowest calorie food items may not be very filling or satisfying. You may need to mix them with food items having more nutrients to produce satiety.

%Ft - Percent of total calories from fat.

The "%Ft" column indicates the percent of the total calories that are fat. Foods high in fat can easily be identified and avoided, and various cooking techniques can be compared to show their effect. For instance, onions are only 3 to 5 percent fat. When creamed, they become 55 percent fat, and when deep fried as onion rings, they become 86 percent fat.

Similar food in various forms can also be compared. Note that skim milk is only 3 percent fat while whole milk is 53 percent. Even 2% milk is fairly high at 38 percent fat, but 1% milk falls into the acceptable range at 18 percent. You may not enjoy skim milk, but most people can learn to like 1% milk. You need to understand that 2% milk is 2 percent fat by weight, but fats provide 38 percent of the total calories. Many foods may appear to be low in fat content when only the relative weight of the fat is listed. For instance, ham is sometimes advertisied as 95 percent fat free, but the total percent of fat is usually over 60 percent.

You will recall that many health authorities are making food recommendations in terms of fat percentage. The Senate Select Committee has recommended a diet containing less than 30 percent fat. More extreme groups recommend diets as low as 10 percent. Our more moderate approach suggests 20 percent fat, with the possibility that some people may need to eat even less. Any food items with a higher fat content than 20 percent need either be avoided, eaten in small quantities, or eaten with other lower fat foods.

P - Protein content in grams (a weight measure).

F - Fat content in grams.

C - Carbohydrate content in grams.

Note: Since alcohol is basically metabolized as a carbohydrate, this guide combines the carbohydrates and alcohols into an equivalent amount of carbohydrate for any alcohol-containing item.

Na - Amount of sodium in milligrams

The last column in the food composition section shows the amount of sodium in milligrams. The main source of sodium is table salt or NaCl, but it is also found in monosodium gluconate, artificial sweeteners like sodium saccharin and in many food additives and drugs. Most health authorities agree that excessive sodium intake is not healthful and may be a major factor in the high incidence of high blood pressure in the modern world. The Senate Select Committee on Nutrition of 1971 recommended that sodium should be restricted to no more than 3200 milligrams daily - about 1/5 of what the average American now eats. Some sodium is found in almost all foods and is absolutely essential for life and good health. You should not restrict sodium to less than 2000 milligrams per day. Under certain circumstances, with high sodium loss like profuse perspiration, some extra sodium may be needed to maintain sodium balance. Those working in very hot conditions may require salt tablets but this is not a problem for most of us.

Sources of Information for Table

This food composition guideline has been prepared from the best sources available. Most of the information came from the United States Department of Agriculture handbook or directly from the manufacturers. Some values are approximate only, but are certainly accurate enough for practical use. Any blank space indicates that the information is not available.

We encourage you to carefully calculate your entire daily food intake at least occasionally. This will help you to learn about foods, about your own diet, and point out areas which require improvement. The optional point system helps with this, but more precise information will be obtained with your complete analysis.

Some food items have a "T" listed under the P, F, or C column. This indicates that there is less then one gram of that particular nutrient.

Calculations Using Food Guidelines

Having access to information about the proportion of various nutrients in a food item makes it easy to calculate the relative amount of that nutrient in each food or even the daily intake of that nutrient. If you wish to calculate the percent of protein in tomatoes, you multiply the number of grams of protein (2) in the tomato by 4, which gives the total calories of protein (since there are 4 calories in each gram of protein). This gives a total of 8 calories of protein compared to the 40 calories total. To find the percentage of calories that are protein calories, divide the protein calories by the total calories and multiply by 100 to express as a percent.

$$\frac{8}{40} \times 100 = 20\%$$

The same type of calculation can be done for carbohydrates or fats. Keep in mind that each gram of protein and carbohydrate has 4 calories, but that each gram of fat has 9 calories.

The main problem with this type of calculation is that some food items are so small and the estimate of nutrient weight is rounded off to the nearest number; thus, a large rounding error can occur. For this reason we calculated the percent of fat from a more detailed source to give more accurate levels. When used for an entire meal or an entire day's eating, the rounding problems tend to average out and a reasonably accurate figure will emerge.

You may find it interesting and informative to calculate the nutrient content for an entire meal or for a whole day. There is a simple way of making the calculation:
- List all foods eaten with a calculation of their calories, protein, fat, and carbohydrate content.
- Add all figures for each column together.
- To calculate fat calories, multiply fat grams by 9. Divide fat calories by the total calories and multiply by 100 to express as a percentage.

• To calculate protein and carbohydrate calories, multiply the total grams of each by 4 (since there are 4 calories in each gram). Divide protein and carbohydrate calories by total calories, and multiply by 100 to express as a percentage. For example, a typical Sunday dinner may look like this:

Foods	Amount	Calories	%Fat	P	F	C	RCU	FU
Roast Beef (rib)	8 oz.	1000	81	46	90	0	0	11
Mashed potatoes	1 cup	125	7	4	1	25	0	0
Butter (potatoes)	1 Tb.	100	99	0	11	0	0	2
Gravy	4 Tb.	100	72	T	8	4	0	2
Creamed Corn	1/2 cup	95	9	2	1	19	0	0
Green toss salad	1 bowl	52	8	4	1	10	0	0
Salad dressing (bleu cheese)	3 Tbs.	267	84	T	27	6	0	3
Apple pie	4″ wedge	350	39	3	15	50	7	2
Ice cream	1 scoop	150	54	3	9	15	2	1
Totals		2239		62	163	129	9	21

Total calories   = 2239
Total protein calories   62 x 4 = 248
Total fat calories   163 x 9 = 1467
Total carbohydrate calories   129 x 4 = 516

Percent Protein   248/2239 x 100 = 11
Percent Fat   1377/2239 x 100 = 66
Percent Carbohydrate 516/2239 x 100 = 23
Total   = 100 percent

    This type of meal is not too different from a typical restaurant meal. Even if you only ate half of each item listed, the ratios and fat percentage would be the same.

    By observing the foods that are high in fat content and reducing them (while increasing the amount of food low in fat) you can greatly improve the situation. Using basically the same food except for the dessert, but with different ratios, your meal would look like this:

Foods	Amount	Calor-ies	%Fat	P	F	C	RCU	FU
Roast beef (rib)	2 oz.	250	81	11	22	0	0	3
Mashed Potatoes (no butter)	2 cups	250	7	8	2	50	0	0
Gravy	2 Tbs.	50	72	T	4	2	0	1
Creamed Corn	1 cup	190	9	4	2	38	0	0
Green Salad	2 bowls	102	8	8	2	20	0	0
Salad Dress-ing (bleu cheese)	1 Tb.	89	69	T	9	2	0	1
Totals		931		31	41	112	0	5
Calories				124	369	448		
Percent of total calories				15	40	48		

Choosing a leaner beef source, a low-fat diet salad dressing, and an apple for dessert, a further improvement can be made:

Foods	Amount	Calo-ries	%Fat	P	F	C	RCU	FU
Tenderloin Steak	2 oz	120	45	17	6	0	0	1
Mashed Potatoes (no butter)	2 cups	250	7	8	2	50	0	0
Gravy	2 Tbs.	50	72	T	4	2	0	1
Creamed Corn	1 cup	190	9	4	2	38	0	0
Green Salad	2 bowls	102	8	8	2	20	0	0
Diet Salad Dressing (bleu cheese)	2 Tb.	26	69	2	2	T	0	0
Apple	1 med.	80	11	T	T	20	0	0
Totals		818	1	39	18	130	0	2
Total Calories				156	162	520		
Percent of Calories				19	20	63		

This example should help you see how easy it is to decrease fat and protein intake with only minor changes. Note that the total volume of food is not too much different from the original dinner which had 62 percent fat and over 2000 calories.

You will note that the Composition of Food Guide gives a good idea of fat content by three different methods.

- The Point System. By getting full points for fat intake your percentage of fats should be very close at 20 percent provided that you are eating adequate calories.

- %Fat column gives the percent of the calories that come from fats for each food item. By completely avoiding most food items over 20 percent fat, by greatly reducing the quantity of the ones that you do get, and by mixing them with other foods lower than 20 percent fat, you can come out fairly close to a 20 percent fat diet without a lot of calculations.
- You can count the fat calories and calculate the percent of fat in any meal or an entire day's eating.

You may be mislead by looking at only one particular comparative measure. For example, if you looked at only percent fat, you will notice that frozen strawberries has only 2 percent fat while fresh strawberries have 12 percent. The difference is that the sweetened strawberries are loaded with sugar, which makes the natural fats in the berries a much smaller percentage of the total calories. You would get the same amount of fat in 1 cup of strawberries whether sweetened or not, but would get much more sugar with the sweetened berries.

COMPOSITION OF FOOD TABLES

Item	Portion	RCU	FU	Cal	RCal	%Ft	P	F	C	Na
Abalone	4 oz.	0	0	100	98	5	21	T	3	
Almonds, dried	12 med.	0	1	100	598	81	3	9	3	1
roasted and salted	12 med.	0	1	105	627	86	3	10	3	33
Anchovies, canned	2 oz.	0	1	100	176	54	11	6	T	
Anchovy paste	2 Tbs.	0	1	100	353	54	10	6	2	3,080
Apple brown betty	4 oz.	3	1	171	151	21	1	4	33	174
Applebutter	1 Tbs.	1	0	35	186	4	T	T	9	T
Apple juice	8 oz.	0	0	110	47	T	T	T	28	2
Apples:										
baked, w/2 Tbs. sugar	1 large	2	0	200	88	1	1	T	47	10
dried, uncooked	4 oz.	0	0	312	275	5	T	T	82	2
dried, cooked, sweetened	1/2 cup	3	0	157	112	3	T	T	41	1
unsweetened	1/2 cup	0	0	100	78	6	T	T	25	1
fresh, peeled	1 med.	0	0	70	54	5	T	T	18	1
fresh, unpeeled	1 med.	0	0	80	58	11	T	T	20	1
Applesauce, sweetened	4 oz.	2	0	100	91	1	T	T	25	3
unsweetened	4 oz.	0	0	55	41	4	T	T	13	2
Apricot nectar	4 oz.	0	0	65	57	2	T	T	17	T
Apricots:										
canned, heavy syrup	4 halves	3	0	105	86	1	1	T	27	1
canned, light syrup	4 oz.	2	0	75	66	1	T	T	19	1
canned, water pack	4 oz.	0	0	40	38	2	T	T	10	1
dried	3 small	0	0	60	260	2	1	T	13	6
fresh, whole	3	0	0	66	51	4	1	T	14	1
Artichoke, boiled, drained	1 avg.	0	0	50	30	6	2	T	10	45

Item	Portion	RCU	FU	Cal	RCal	%Ft	P	F	C	Na
Artichoke hearts, frozen	3	0	0	22	41	9	1	T	5	0
Asparagus:										
boiled	6 spears	0	0	20	22	9	2	T	3	1
canned, drained	6 spears	0	0	20	21	17	2	T	3	227
frozen	4 oz.	0	0	25	22	9	3	T	4	2
Avacado, raw	1/2 avg.	0	2	190	167	85	2	18	7	4
Bacon, Canadian	2 oz.	0	1	155	277	58	16	10	T	1,430
Bacon, crisp	3 strips	0	1	100	611	78	5	8	T	163
Bacon fat	1 tsp.	0	1	50	771	97	1	5	T	40
Baking powder	1 tsp.	0	0	6	129	T	T	T	1	386
Bamboo shoots	4 oz.	0	0	30	27	9	3	T	5	
Banana	1 med.	0	0	95	85	2	1	T	23	1
Barbecue Sauce	1 Tbs.	0	1	50	91	90	2	5	T	200
Barley	4 oz.	0	0	390	349	2	9	1	88	5
Bass, baked & stuffed	4 oz.	0	2	280	259	58	18	18	12	100
Bass, fried	4 oz.	0	1	230	202	39	25	10	9	80
Bean sprouts, mung	4 oz.	0	0	40	35	5	4	T	7	5
Bean Sprouts, soy	4 oz.	0	0	115	35	39	8	5	8	5
Beans, baked:										
w/pork & molasses, canned	4 oz.	1	1	170	150	26	7	5	30	430
w/pork & tomato sauce	4 oz.	0	0	140	122	19	7	3	24	525
w/tomato sauce	4 oz.	0	0	135	120	4	8	T	24	379
Beans, green:										
canned	1 cup	0	0	30	24	4	2	T	6	536
fresh, cooked	1 cup	0	0	30	25	7	2	T	6	8
frozen or raw	4 oz.	0	0	40	25	6	2	T	8	8
Beans, kidney, cooked	1 cup	0	0	225	118	4	14	T	37	6
Beans, lima:										
canned, drained	4 oz.	0	0	80	46	3	4	T	15	205
dried	4 oz.	0	0	391	345	4	23	1	69	4
fresh	4 oz.	0	0	135	111	4	8	T	27	2
Beans, pinto, raw	1/2 cup	0	0	390	339	2	25	1	72	10
cooked, no salt	1 cup	0	0	266	116	4	15	1	49	15
Beans, wax, canned, drained	4 oz.	0	0	30	244	11	2	T	5	146
fresh, boiled	4 oz.	0	0	30	22	8	2	T	5	3
Beef, cooked:										
broiled, lean meat only	4 oz.	0	2	254	224	43	34	12	0	68
broiled, lean meat and fat	4 oz.	0	6	528	465	82	22	48	0	68
chuck (pot roast)	4 oz.	0	3	372	327	66	30	27	0	68
corned	4 oz.	0	4	423	372	73	26	35	0	1,973
dried	3 oz.	0	1	175	203	28	29	5	0	3,526
fillet mignon (broiled)	4 oz.	0	6	516	454	80	23	46	0	68
flank, braised	4 oz.	0	1	223	196	33	35	8	0	68
ground beef (hamburger), lean	4 oz.	0	2	248	219	47	31	13	0	55
ground beef (hamburger), regular	4 oz.	0	3	325	285	64	27	23	0	53
heart, lean	4 oz.	0	1	213	188	25	36	6	0	104
Jerky	1 oz.	0	1	100	352	25	16	3	0	812
kidney, braised	4 oz.	0	2	285	252	43	37	14	1	288
liver, fried	4 oz.	0	2	260	229	42	30	12	6	210
rib roast	4 oz.	0	6	500	440	81	23	45	0	68
round steak	4 oz.	0	2	296	261	53	32	17	0	68

Item	Portion	RCU	FU	Cal	RCal	%Ft	P	F	C	Na
short ribs, braised	4 oz.	0	2	200	176	54	23	12	0	68
sirloin tip	4 oz.	0	5	439	387	75	26	36	0	68
suet	1 oz.	0	4	240	854	98	T	26	0	0
sweetbreads	2 avg.	0	2	160	141	68	13	12	0	58
tenderloin steak	4 oz.	0	2	240	211	45	34	12	0	68
tongue	4 oz.	0	2	225	198	68	19	17	T	70
Beef Pot Pie, baked	4″ dia.	2	4	527	192	53	22	31	40	607
Beef stew, fresh	4 oz.	0	1	100	88	45	7	5	7	45
Beer (see beverages)										
Beet greens	1 cup	0	0	25	18	11	2	T	4	105
Beets, raw	4 oz.	0	0	50	43	2	2	T	10	70
Beets, canned	4 oz.	0	0	35	37	2	1	T	8	236
Beverages:										
Beer	12 oz.	6	0	151	42	0	1	0	37*	25
Lite Beer	12 oz.	4	0	96	28	0	1	0	23*	T
Cocktails:										
w/club soda or tomato juice	5 fl. oz.	6	0	200	141	T	1	T	47*	200
Pina Colada	3 fl. oz.	10	0	240	282	T	T	T	60*	2
Other mixed drinks	5 fl. oz.	6	0	132	93	T	T	T	33*	2
Distilled Liquors (Gin, Rum, Vodka, Whiskey)										
80 proof	2 fl. oz.	5	0	130	231	0	0	0	32*	1
86 proof	2 fl. oz.	6	0	140	249	0	0	0	36*	1
90 proof	2 fl. oz.	6	0	148	263	0	0	0	38*	1
94 proof	2 fl. oz.	7	0	154	275	0	0	0	39*	1
100 proof	2 fl. oz.	7	0	166	295	0	0	0	42*	1
Wine:										
Cooking sherry	4 oz.	2	0	38	34	0	0	0	10*	660
Dessert (18.8% alcohol)	4 oz.	7	0	163	138	0	0	0	41*	5
Table (12.2% alcohol)	4 oz.	4	0	100	85	0	0	0	25*	5
Milk:										
skimmed	1 cup	0	0	85	37	3	9	T	13	123
whole	1 cup	0	1	170	66	53	9	10	8	131
Orange juice	1 cup	0	0	110	49	4	2	T	26	2
Soft drinks, Diet	12 oz.	0	0	1	0	0	0	0	T	60
Soft drinks, regular	12 oz.	7	0	157	66	0	0	0	38	T
V-8 Vegetable juice	1 cup	0	0	45	20	4	2	T	9	872
Water	1 cup	0	0	0	0	0	0	0	0	2
Big Mac Hamburger	1	3	4	541		52	26	31	39	962
Biscuit, baking powder	1 2″ dia.	1	1	103	370	44	2	5	12	175
Blackberries	1 cup	0	0	60	58	7	1	T	13	1
Blackberry juice	1 cup	0	0	80	37	15	1	T	19	2
Black-eyed peas, cowpeas	4 oz.	0	0	83	70	4	6	T	14	33
Blueberries, canned, sweetened	1 cup	1	0	100	105	6	T	T	26	1
Blueberries, fresh	1 cup	0	0	60	62	11	T	T	17	1
Bologna	2 oz.	0	2	165	304	76	8	14	T	705
Bouillion cube	1	0	0	5	120	18	T	T	0	400
Boysenberries:										
canned	4 oz.	0	0	40	36	2	T	T	10	1
fresh	1 cup	0	0	60	48	1	T	T	13	1

Item	Portion	RCU	FU	Cal	RCal	%Ft	P	F	C	Na
frozen, sweetened	4 oz.	2	0	110	96	3	T	T	27	1
frozen, unsweetened	4 oz.	0	0	55	48	1	T	T	14	1
Bran, wheat	1 oz.	0	0	60	211	15	5	1	8	3
Brazilnuts	2 oz.	0	4	365	654	86	8	35	6	1
Bread:										
Boston brown	1 slice	2	0	105	211	9	2	1	24	124
Cracked wheat	1 slice	1	0	60	263	8	2	T	12	121
Fresh Horizons	1 slice	1	0	54		7	3	T	10	
Hollywood	1 slice	1	0	49		7	2	T	9	
French	1 slice	1	0	50	290	9	2	T	10	100
Italian	1 slice	1	0	60	276	3	2	T	12	127
pumpernickel	1 slice	1	0	70	246	4	2	T	16	182
raisin	1 slice	1	0	65	262	10	2	T	12	91
rye	1 slice	0	0	75	243	4	2	T	12	172
Vienna	1 slice	1	0	60	290	15	2	1	10	133
white	1 slice	1	0	65	269	12	2	T	12	122
whole wheat	1 slice	0	0	65	269	11	3	T	11	141
Bread, sweet:										
banana nut	1 slice	2	0	185	592	10	3	2	22	212
date nut	1 slice	2	0	100	320	9	2	1	21	155
Bread sticks, Vienna type	1 oz.	1	0	86	304	10	T	T	16	444
Bread Stuffing Mix	1/2 cup	2	0	118	371	8	4	1	26	647
Breadcrumbs, dry, grated	1 Tbs.	0	0	25	392	11	T	T	5	47
Broccoli, fresh	4 oz.	0	0	30	32	9	3	T	5	15
Broccoli, frozen	4 oz.	0	0	35	28	10	4	T	6	15
Brussel sprouts, cooked	1 cup	0	0	50	36	9	5	T	9	15
Bulgur, canned, seasoned	1 cup	2	1	246	168	16	8	5	44	621
Butter, salted	1 Tbs.	0	2	100	716	99	T	11	T	138
unsalted	1 Tbs.	0	2	100	716	99	T	11	T	2
Buttermilk	1 cup	0	0	85	36	3	T	T	12	307
Butterfish, northern raw	4 oz.	0	1	190	169	52	20	11	0	12
Cabbage, boiled	1/2 cup	0	0	16	20	9	1	T	3	12
Cabbage, Chinese	4 oz.	0	0	15	14	7	1	T	3	24
Cabbage, coleslaw	4 oz.	0	1	110	99	74	1	9	7	125
Skipper's coleslaw	1 serving	1	5	377	144	86	3	36	11	314
Cabbage, raw, shredded	1 cup	0	0	25	24	7	1	T	5	20
Cakes:										
angel food	1/12	4	0	135	269	1	3	T	32	142
applesauce	3 oz.	7	2	400	352	27	4	12	63	368
cheese cake, graham-										
cracker crust	1/8 cake	8	4	510	397	45	5	25	57	347
chocolate, iced	4 oz.	7	1	345	369	23	3	9	64	220
coconut (Duncan Hines)	1/12	3	1	200		32	3	7	29	377
cupcake, iced (1.8 oz.)	1	3	1	184	369	29	2	6	30	168
devils food	2 oz.	4	1	210	369	34	2	8	32	162
fruitcake, dark, 2"x2"x1/2"	1	2	1	114	379	32	2	4	18	47
poundcake, 1/2" slice	1	2	1	140	473	57	2	9	14	33
upside-down	1/9	4	1	275	390	33	7	10	38	360
yellow	1/16	4	1	200	363	32	2	7	32	134
white	1/16	5	1	250	375	29	3	8	45	161
Candy:										
almond chocolate bar	1 oz.	3	1	150	569	60	1	10	17	22
almonds/choc. Estee diet	3/4 oz.	2	1	125	569	65	2	9	9	28

Item	Portion	RCU	FU	Cal	RCal	%Ft	P	F	C	Na
butterscotch	1 oz.	4	1	120	397	23	1	3	24	94
carmel	1 med.	1	1	60	399	45	1	3	8	34
chocolate, bitter or baking	1 oz.	1	3	145	477	93	3	15	8	1
milk, semi-sweet	1 oz.	3	2	145	507	6	2	9	16	26
fondant	1 oz.	4	0	105	410	9	T	1	25	61
fudge	1 oz.	4	1	120	400	30	1	4	21	57
gum drops	1 oz.	4	0	100	347	T	T	T	25	10
hard candies	1 oz.	5	0	110	386	T	0	T	28	9
Estee assorted	1 oz.	5	0	113	396	T	0	T	28	5
jelly beans	1 oz.	4	0	104	367	0	T	0	26	3
marshmallows	1 avg.	1	0	25	319	0	T	0	6	3
peanut brittle (no salt)	1 oz.	4	1	120	421	23	T	3	23	9
raisins, chocolate covered	1 oz.	3	1	120	425	30	2	4	20	18
raisins, Estee Choc. covered	1 oz.	2	1	140	490	51	3	8	14	28
Candy bars:										
Almond Joy	1 oz.	2	1	132	462	48	1	7	16	40
BabyRuth	1 oz.	4	1	135	473	33	1	5	21	100
Butterfinger	1 oz.	4	1	134	469	33	1	5	21	93
Caravelle	1 oz.	3	1	127	445	35	1	5	19	50
Kisses, Herseys	1 piece	1	0	25	528	36	T	1	4	5
Licorice, black	1 oz.	3	0	100	350	18	T	2	20	30
Life Savers	5 pieces	2	0	45	386	0	0	T	10	5
Mars Bar	1 oz.	2	1	130	455	48	T	7	17	56
Mint Pattie	1 piece	2	0	50	410	18	T	1	10	3
M & M's	1 oz.	3	1	140	490	45	2	7	18	5
Peanut Butter Cup	1 oz.	3	1	143	501	44	2	7	15	99
Snickers	1 oz.	3	1	130	455	55	T	8	15	100
3 Musketeers	1 oz.	3	1	120	420	30	T	4	20	20
Toffee	1 piece	1	0	28	400	32	T	1	5	90
Cantaloupe	1/4 melon	0	0	35	30	T	1	T	8	14
Carnation Instant Breakfast										
with skim milk	1 cup	4	0	387	170	7	15	3	35	415
Carrots, raw	1 cup	0	0	45	30	4	1	T	10	50
canned	1 cup	0	0	45	30	6	1	T	10	354
frozen	1 cup	0	0	50	30	5	T	T	10	28
Casaba melon	1/2 lb.	0	0	31	30	3	T	T	8	13
Cashew nuts, salted	2 oz.	0	3	335	561	70	10	26	16	119
unsalted	2 oz.	0	3	335	561	70	10	26	16	9
Catsup, regular pack	1 Tbs.	0	0	15	106	3	T	T	4	147
low sodium	1 Tbs.	0	0	15	106	3	T	T	4	4
Cauliflower, raw or boiled	1 cup	0	0	30	27	7	3	T	5	14
frozen	1 cup	0	0	50	18	9	4	T	8	18
Celery, raw	1 cup	0	0	20	17	6	1	T	5	151
cooked	1 cup	0	0	21	14	T	1	T	5	132
Cereal:										
All Bran	1/2 cup	0	0	64	224	14	3	1	11	287
Alpha Bits	1 cup	3	0	113	50	8	2	1	24	150
Apple Jacks	1 cup	3	0	110	48	3	1	T	26	68
Barley, dry	1 oz.	0	0	100	350	3	2	T	22	1
Bran Buds	1/3 cup	0	0	73	256	12	3	1	13	63
40% Bran Flakes	1/2 cup	1	0	87	303	2	3	T	23	162
100% Bran	1/2 cup	1	0	97	340	5	3	1	19	187

Item	Portion	RCU	FU	Cal	RCal	%Ft	P	F	C	Na
Buc Wheats	1 cup	1	0	102	359	9	3	1	20	264
Cheerios	1 cup	1	0	112	395	T	2	T	26	256
Corn Chex	1 1/4 cup	1	0	111	392	T	2	T	26	304
Cornflakes	1 cup	1	0	95	386	T	2	T	21	201
Cream of Wheat, regular	3/4 cup	0	0	100	42	9	4	1	21	1
Farina, cooked	1 cup	0	0	100	42	9	4	1	21	1
Granola, Nature Valley	1/3 cup	2	1	150	528	36	6	6	18	218
Grape Nuts	1/4 cup	1	0	104	367	1	3	T	22	147
Grape Nuts Flakes	2/3 cup	1	0	107	377	2	3	T	22	150
Kix	1 cup	1	0	120	399	8	2	1	25	330
Life	1 cup	1	0	160	377	11	5	2	30	264
Malt-O-Meal	3/4 cup	0	0	102	44	9	3	1	22	1
Maypo, Instant	1 oz.	1	0	107	377	9	4	1	21	1
Natural Cereal, Quaker	1/4 cup	1	1	140	245	39	3	6	19	19
Oat Flakes, Post	2/3 cup	1	0	107	377	8	5	1	20	198
Oatmeal, cooked, instant	3/4 cup	0	0	107	69	17	4	2	18	255
regular	1 cup	0	0	150	55	18	5	3	25	1
Pep	3/4 cup	1	0	100	353	2	2	T	24	184
Product 19	3/4 cup	1	0	110	388	1	3	T	24	271
Puffed Oats	1 oz.	0	0	113	399	8	3	1	22	359
Puffed Rice	1 cup	0	0	55	388	2	1	T	14	1
Puffed Wheat	1 cup	0	0	54	381	3	2	T	11	1
Raisin Bran	1/2 cup	1	0	102	360	2	3	T	22	190
Rice Chex	1 cup	0	0	98	388	1	2	T	22	228
Rice Flakes, puffed	1/2 cup	0	0	55	399	1	1	T	13	198
Roman Meal	3/4 cup	0	0	130	91	7	5	1	25	2
Shredded Wheat	1 oz.	0	0	105	354	9	3	1	23	1
Special K	1 cup	0	0	87	388	10	3	1	17	134
Sugared Prepared Cereals	3/4 cup	2	0	110	388	3	1	T	26	200
Total	1 cup	1	0	110	388	8	2	1	23	48
Wheat, rolled, uncooked	1 cup	0	0	296	340	6	9	2	60	2
cooked with salt	1 cup	0	0	163	75	5	5	1	34	640
Wheaties	1 cup	1	0	110	388	8	2	1	23	314
Whole Bran	1/2 cup	0	0	60	211	15	5	1	8	187
Cheese:										
American	1 oz.	0	1	105	377	73	6	9	T	322
Bleu	1 oz.	0	1	104	368	74	6	9	T	510
Cheddar	1 oz.	0	1	113	398	72	7	9	T	198
Cottage, creamed	1 oz.	0	0	30	106	36	4	1	1	65
With skim milk	1 oz.	0	0	25	86	4	5	T	1	84
Cream	1 oz.	0	1	106	374	91	2	11	T	71
Edam	1 oz.	0	1	125	441	94	9	13	2	204
Monterey Jack	1 oz.	0	1	102	360	71	8	8	T	204
Mozzarella	1 oz.	0	1	84	317	75	5	7	T	227
Parmesan, dry grated	1 oz.	0	1	105	393	60	10	7	T	247
Roquefort	1 oz.	0	1	105	368	69	6	8	T	465
Swiss	1 oz.	0	1	105	370	69	6	8	T	201
Velveeta	1 oz.	0	1	105	370	69	6	8	T	554
Cheese Fondue	4 oz.	0	3	315	265	60	20	21	9	615
Cheese Omelet	2 eggs	0	3	260	218	73	18	21	1	434
Cheese sauce from mix	1/2 cup	0	2	225	149	72	11	18	5	989
Cheese souffle	1/2 cup	0	2	240	218	71	11	19	6	400
Cheese spreads	1 oz.	0	1	82	288	66	5	6	2	461

Item	Portion	RCU	FU	Cal	RCal	%Ft	P	F	C	Na
Cherries:										
sweet in light syrup	1 cup	1	0	90	65	4	1	T	19	1
sour in light syrup	1 cup	1	0	100	74	3	1	T	24	1
fresh	1 cup	0	0	85	70	4	1	T	20	2
maraschino	2	0	0	10	116	T	T	T	2	
Chestnuts, dried	8 med.	0	0	50	377	18	1	1	11	1
Chestnuts, fresh	4 oz.	2	0	220	194	8	3	2	47	7
Chicken:										
a la king	4 oz.	0	2	215	191	67	14	16	4	349
barbecued or broiled	4 oz.	0	2	225	198	56	23	14	T	310
creamed	4 oz.	0	3	385	340	61	32	26	6	706
Fryer - baked:										
all flesh with skin	4 oz.	0	1	181	159	34	26	6	0	98
dark meat with skin	4 oz.	0	1	189	166	40	25	7	0	98
dark meat	4 oz.	0	1	160	141	25	25	4	0	98
light meat with skin	4 oz.	0	1	172	151	27	28	5	0	90
light meat	4 oz.	0	0	144	127	12	28	2	0	73
Fryer - fried:										
dark meat with skin	4 oz.	0	2	299	263	47	34	15	0	90
dark meat	4 oz.	0	1	249	220	38	35	11	0	88
light meat with skin	4 oz.	0	1	266	234	38	36	11	0	75
light meat	4 oz.	0	1	224	197	28	36	7	0	68
Kentucky Fried, Original	1 piece	2	2	227		59	17	15	19	762
giblets, raw	4 oz.	0	0	105	93	26	19	3	T	74
giblets, fried	4 oz.	0	2	270	252	40	35	12	5	80
livers, cooked	4 oz.	0	1	185	163	24	30	5	2	69
livers, paste	1 oz.	0	2	145	511	87	3	14	2	50
Chicken pie	4 oz.	1	2	225	199	52	7	13	20	245
Chickpeas, dry uncooked	4 oz.	0	0	390	360	12	23	5	60	28
Chip beef	2 oz.	0	1	110	203	32	19	4	0	2,330
Chili with beans	1 cup	0	2	335	133	40	19	15	30	1,337
Chili without beans	1 cup	0	5	510	200	67	26	38	15	1,693
Chili Bowl, Wendy's	1 serving	0	1	230	135	31	19	8	21	1,065
Chili powder	1 tsp.	0	0	17	340	0	0	0	4	79
Chili sauce	1 Tbs.	0	0	17	21	T	0	T	4	201
Chives	1 oz.	0	0	5	28	T	T	T	1	T
Chop Suey:										
chicken or pork	1 cup	0	1	120	48	45	5	6	12	1,067
beef, canned	1 cup	0	1	155	62	46	11	8	10	1,378
vegetable	1 cup	0	1	112	45	48	4	6	11	995
Chow Mein:										
beef, canned	4 oz.	0	3	275	242	65	20	20	4	1,080
chicken or pork	4 oz.	0	1	115	102	31	14	4	4	323
Cider, apple	1 cup	0	0	100	47	T	T	T	25	2
Citron, candied	2 oz.	6	0	180	314	1	T	T	45	166
Clams:										
broiled	6	0	1	115		47	10	6	5	181
canned, drained	4 oz.	0	0	105	98	26	17	3	2	166
cherrystone	6	0	0	100		18	15	2	5	157
fried	6	0	1	200	311	68	12	15	5	525
raw	4 oz.	0	0	90	52	20	15	2	4	142
roasted	6	0	1	135		40	15	6	5	213

Item	Portion	RCU	FU	Cal	RCal	%Ft	P	F	C	Na
Skipper's Clams	1 serving	1	3	434		56	14	27	33	358
steamed	4 oz.	0	0	100	67	27	12	3	4	157
Clam Chowder, Skipper's	1 cup	0	0	102	45	35	4	4	12	1,055
Cocktail sauce	1 oz.	0	0	31	109	T	0	T	8	340
Cocoa, with skimmed milk	1 cup	2	0	130	57	T	8	T	26	190
with whole milk	1 cup	2	1	165	73	38	7	7	18	161
Cocoa syrup	1 Tbs.	2	0	40	245	7	T	T	12	110
Coconut:										
fresh	2 oz.	0	3	210	346	86	2	20	11	14
dried, lightly packed,										
sweetened	1/2 cup	3	2	252	548	64	2	18	21	136
unsweetened	1/2 cup	0	4	305	662	89	3	30	6	25
Coconut milk (commercial)	4 oz.	0	3	286	252	85	4	27	5	132
Codfish, broiled	4 oz.	0	1	180	170	30	32	6	0	116
Codfish cakes, fried	4 oz.	0	1	195	172	47	16	9	11	130
Coffee:										
black	1 cup	0	0	2	1	T	T	T	T	2
with cream	1 cup	0	0	30	13	90	T	3	1	8
with cream and sugar	1 cup	1	0	50	22	54	T	3	5	8
Coleslaw - see cabbage										
Collards	1/2 cup	0	0	45	45	40	2	2	5	43
Cookies:										
Animal crackers	6	1	0	50	430	18	1	1	12	72
Arrowroot	1	0	0	25	500	36	T	1	4	12
Brownies	1 oz.	2	1	119	485	61	2	8	17	
Butterscotch	1	2	1	140	481	51	3	8	15	161
Chocolate chip	3 med.	2	1	150	515	36	2	6	22	115
Chocolate wafers	1	1	0	40	445	23	2	1	6	29
Coconut macaroons	2 small	2	1	100	494	45	3	5	14	42
Fig Newton	2	2	0	100	358	9	1	1	22	193
Ginger snaps	5	1	1	165	420	55	1	10	6	224
Graham Crackers	3 med.	1	0	75	357	24	1	2	15	141
Oatmeal	1 large	1	0	90	451	30	2	3	15	76
Peanut	1	1	0	65	473	28	1	2	9	24
Scotch shortbread	1	0	0	35	498	51	T	2	5	4
Sugar	1 med.	1	0	50	444	36	1	2	7	36
Vanilla Wafer	1	1	0	25	462	36	T	1	4	14
Cool Whip topping	1/3 cup	1	1	84	334	64	0	5	5	11
Corn:										
boiled, fresh on the cob	1 small	0	0	75	91	12	3	1	17	T
cream style	1/2 cup	0	0	95	82	9	2	1	19	273
niblets	1/2 cup	0	0	95	83	9	3	1	18	318
Corn chips	1 oz.	0	1	164	577	60	1	11	15	160
Corn grits, cooked	1/2 cup	0	0	55	51	1	1	T	14	221
Cornbread	2 oz.	1	1	170	207	26	4	5	22	516
Cornmeal	1/2 cup	3	0	230	355	8	5	2	45	1
Cornstarch	1 Tbs.	0	0	30	362	30	1	1	7	T
Crab Meat:										
canned	3 oz.	0	0	85	101	21	15	2	1	842
frozen	1/2 cup	0	0	70	93	26	13	2	T	1
Crabapples	1 large	0	0	90	68	T	1	T	21	1
Cracker meal	2 oz.	4	1	265	439	27	6	8	42	664
Crackers:										

Item	Portion	RCU	FU	Cal	RCal	%Ft	P	F	C	Na
Bacon Thins	8 pieces	1	1	88	550	55	T	5	10	256
Bugles, General Mills	15 pieces	1	1	150	529	49	2	8	17	138
Butter Thins, Nabisco	10 pieces	2	1	150	467	60	2	5	24	160
Cheese cracker, Kraft										
4 crackers & 3/4 oz.										
cheese	1 packet	1	0	138	433	8	1	1	31	68
Cheese Nips, Nabisco	24 pieces	1	1	114	401	55	4	7	15	422
Cheez-Its, Sunshine	10 pieces	1	0	60	600	45		1	3	7
Cheese Ritz	10 pieces	2	1	170	567	53	3	9	19	350
Che-Tos, fried	2 oz.	1	1	150	266	42	1	9	17	220
Cheese & Peanut										
butter square	4 pieces	1	1	141	491	45	4	7	15	332
Chicken in a Biskit, Nab.	10 pieces	1	1	110	550	82	5	5	11	190
Club, Keebler	10 pieces	2	1	150	500	60	2	7	20	440
Corn chips, Fritos, regular	1 oz.	1	1	159	561	62	2	11	13	160
barbecued	1 oz.	1	1	159	561	62	2	11	13	190
Corn Diggers, Nabisco	20 pieces	1	1	80	444	45	2	4	9	200
Goldfish, Pepperidge Farm	20 pieces	1	0	58	493	31	T	2	10	164
Pretzel	20 pieces	1	0	58	409	31	2	2	8	390
Graham	4 squares	2	0	110	386	22	2	3	21	190
Sugar-honey coated	4 squares	2	0	116	413	25	2	3	21	144
Hi-Ho, Sunshine	10 pieces	2	1	180	590	50	2	10	20	350
Onion flavored:										
French, Nabisco	10 pieces	1	1	120	600	38	2	5	15	310
Toast, Keebler	10 pieces	2	1	180	599	35	T	1	2	290
Oyster	10 pieces	1	0	44	437	27	1	1	9	110
Peanut butter Sandwich	6 pieces	2	1	201	414	39	4	9	26	493
Pizza Spins, General Mills	32 pieces	1	1	150	529	24	2	4	15	218
Ritz	8 pieces	2	1	136	567	52	1	8	32	256
Rye Toast, Keebler	10 toasts	1	1	170	425	53	3	8	22	390
Ry-Krisp	5 pieces	0	0	120	400	4	4	1	25	375
Saltine	5 squares	1	0	61	428	25	1	2	10	156
Sesame Buttery, Nabisco	10 pieces	2	1	165	550	44	3	8	20	350
Sociables, Nabisco	10 pieces	1	1	100	500	36	2	4	13	300
Soda	5 squares	2	1	120	439	36	3	4	18	300
Tortilla chips, Doritos	1 oz.	0	1	137	483	40	2	6	19	130
Taco flavor	1 oz.	0	1	140	494	39	2	6	19	240
Triangle Thins, Nabisco	10 pieces	1	0	80	400	34	2	3	11	240
Triscuit, Nabisco	10 pieces	2	1	210	525	34	4	8	31	300
Waldorf, low sodium	10 pieces	2	1	140	467	26	3	4	23	9
Waverly Wafer, Nabisco	10 pieces	2	1	180	450	40	2	8	25	460
Wheat Thins, Nabisco	10 pieces	1	1	90	450	40	1	4	13	230
Wheatsworth	9 pieces	1	1	130	458	42	3	6	16	150
Zwieback	5 pieces	2	1	155	423	20	5	4	25	30
Cranberries	4 oz.	0	0	52	46	14	T	T	11	2
Cranberry juice cocktail	4 oz.	1	0	75	65	1	T	T	18	1
Cranberry sauce, jellied	1 Tbs.	1	0	50	146	1	T	T	13	T
Cranberry relish	1 Tbs.	1	0	65	178	2	T	T	15	T
Cream:										
Half & Half	1/2 cup	0	2	160	134	79	4	13	5	55
Heavy	1 Tbs.	0	1	50	352	96	T	5	T	5
Light	1/2 cup	0	3	235	211	88	2	23	5	28
Sour	2 Tbs.	0	1	61	211	89	1	5	1	10

Item	Portion	RCU	FU	Cal	RCal	%Ft	P	F	C	Na
Imitation non-dairy (Pet)	2 Tbs.	0	1	61	176	89	1	6	1	32
Cream sauce, white, medium	2 Tbs.	0	1	50	161	72	3	4	2	117
Creamer, non-dairy	1 tsp.	0	0	11	508	59	T	1	1	11
Croutons	12 avg.	1	1	70	466	51	4	4	6	176
Cucumber	8 inch	0	0	15	15	0	T	0	3	6
Currants, dried (Del Monte)	1/2 cup	2	0	204	300	1	2	T	48	20
fresh	2 oz.	0	0	30	50	1	1	T	5	2
Croissant Rolls (1.5 oz.)	1 tiny	4	1	254	596	35	4	10	36	
Dandelion greens, cooked	4 oz.	0	0	40	33	16	2	T	8	53
Danish pastry	2 oz.	3	1	240	422	49	4	13	25	208
Dates, dried, pitted	1/2 cup	2	0	280	274	1	2	T	65	1
Dips:										
Nalley's Bacon & Onion	1 oz.	0	1	114	402	87	2	11	1	201
Blue Cheese, clam or onion	1 oz.	0	1	106	374	85	2	10	1	175
Doughnut, plain	1 oz.	1	1	120	414	53	1	7	13	102
iced	1 oz.	2	1	127	409	50	1	7	14	205
Duck, roasted	4 oz.	0	1	190	193	43	22	9	0	75
Eclair, chocolate custard	1	2	2	240	239	56	7	15	20	82
Eggs:										
boiled or poached	1	0	1	80	163	68	6	6	T	133
deviled	2	0	3	225	230	60	20	15	2	244
fried	1	0	1	95	216	76	6	8	T	149
scrambled	2	0	2	160	173	68	12	12	T	230
Egg white	1	0	0	10	51	0	3	0	T	29
Egg yolk	1	0	1	70	348	77	3	6	T	12
Eggnog, 6% fat	1/2 cup	3	1	174	133	52	3	10	18	80
Eggplant, boiled	1 cup	0	0	38	19	9	1	T	8	6
Elderberries, whole	1/2 pound	0	0	154	72	1	T	T	36	0
Endive or escarole	8 oz.	0	0	50	20	5	7	T	9	35
Fast Foods:										
Arby's Roast Beef, 5 oz.	1	3	2	350	247	39	22	15	32	880
Arby's Beef & Cheese, 6 oz.	1	3	3	450	265	44	27	22	36	1,220
Arby's Super Roast Beef, 9 oz	1	5	4	620	243	41	30	28	61	1,420
Arby's Jr. Roast Beef, 3 oz.	1	2	1	220	259	37	12	9	21	530
Arby's Ham N Cheese, 5.5 oz.	1	3	2	380	244	40	23	17	33	1,350
Arby's Turkey Deluxe, 8.5 oz.	1	4	3	510	212	42	28	24	46	1,220
Arby's Club, 9 oz.	1	4	4	560	219	48	30	30	43	1,610
Burger King Whopper	1	4	5	630		51	26	36	50	990
Burger King French Fries	1 serving	0	1	210		47	3	11	25	230
Burger King Vanilla Shake	1	7	1	340		29	8	11	52	320
McDonald's Big Mac	1	3	4	541	265	52	26	31	39	962
McDonald's Filet-O-Fish	1	3	3	432		48	15	23	37	709
McDonald's Egg McMuffin	1	2	3	352		51	18	20	26	914
McDonald's Chocolate shake	1	8	1	364		22	11	9	60	329
McDonald's apple pie	1	2	2	253	297	53	1	15	29	414
Pizza Hut Thin'n Crispy, Cheese, 13"	1/2	4	1	340		29	19	11	42	900
Thick'n Chewey, pepperoni 10"	1/2	4	2	450		32	25	16	52	900

Item	Portion	RCU	FU	Cal	RCal	%Ft	P	F	C	Na
Taco Time Burrito, Meat	1	2	2	291		43	20	14	23	848
Soft Bean	1	3	2	341		34	13	13	36	762
Taco Time Soft Flour Taco	1	2	2	296		43	19	14	24	686
Supreme	1	2	3	356		51	19	20	24	696
Taco Time Taco	1	1	1	195		42	14	9	14	591
Fennel Leaves	1 oz.	0	0	9	28	T	1	T	2	0
Figs:										
canned	4 oz.	0	0	75	65	4	T	T	19	4
dried	4	2	0	232	274	1	4	T	52	7
fresh	4 small	0	0	100	80	3	1	T	24	2
Filbert nuts	2 oz.	0	4	365	634	84	8	34	6	1
Finnan haddie	4 oz.	0	0	115	103	11	26	1	0	90
Fish balls	4 oz.	1	1	200	227	45	18	10	7	130
Fish cakes, fried	4 oz.	1	1	190	172	43	16	9	10	130
Fish fillet, Skipper's	1 serving	1	3	277		65	16	20	16	252
Flounder, raw	4 oz.	0	0	90	79	T	18	T	0	106
baked with butter (2 fillets)	4 oz.	0	1	228	201	36	34	9	0	268
Flour:										
All purpose	1 cup	7	0	400	364	2	12	1	84	2
Bisquick	1 cup	7	2	503	222	30	9	17	79	1,476
corn meal	1 cup	4	1	460	368	8	11	4	90	2
rye, dark	1 cup	3	0	410	327	7	20	3	76	1
rye, light	1 cup	4	0	440	357	2	11	1	98	1
self rising, sifted & spooned	1 cup	7	0	373	352	2	10	1	81	1,144
self rising, spooned	1 cup	8	0	447	352	2	12	1	98	1,370
soy bean, defatted	1 cup	1	0	313	326	17	38	6	32	1
whole wheat	1 cup	0	0	350	333	5	14	2	75	3
Frankfurters										
7/8" x 5" (2 oz.)	1	0	2	176	310	80	7	16	1	125
3/4" x 5" (1.6 oz.)	1	0	2	139	310	80	6	12	1	99
Tyson Chicken	1	0	1	120	309	83	5	11	T	427
Fruit cocktail, canned	1 cup	5	0	190	60	1	1	T	47	26
fresh	1 cup	0	0	75	35	2	T	T	19	3
Fruit punch	1 cup	8	0	180	31	T	T	T	45	7
Garlic Clove	1	0	0	5	137	T	1	T	T	1
Gelatin:										
D-Zerta, dietetic	1/2 cup	0	0	8	7	T	2	T	T	6
Knox, powder	1 envelope	0	0	28	335	0	7	0	T	0
Jell-O regular flavors	1/2 cup	3	0	81	59	T	2	T	18	46
wild flavors	1/2 cup	3	0	81	59	T	2	T	18	64
Jells Best, all flavor	1/2 cup	3	0	80	59	0	1	0	19	23
Royal, all flavors	1/2 cup	3	0	82	59	T	2	T	19	90
Goose, Roasted	4 oz.	0	5	480	233	77	27	41	0	255
Gooseberries	1 cup	0	0	60	39	5	T	T	15	2
Grape juice	1 cup	0	0	150	66	T	T	T	37	2
Grapes	1 cup	0	0	95	69	19	2	2	17	4
Grapefruit, fresh	1/2	0	0	50	41	5	1	T	11	1
Grapefruit sections, canned	1/2 cup	0	0	75	30	2	T	T	18	10
Grapefruit juice	1 cup	0	0	90	41	2	1	T	21	2
Gravy	2 Tbs.	0	1	50	88	72	T	4	2	93
Guava	1 med.	0	0	50	62	T	T	T	11	3
Gum, chewing, regular	1 stick	0	0	8	317	0	0	0	2	T
Diet, Carefree	1 stick	0	0	7	277	0	0	0	2	T

Item	Portion	RCU	FU	Cal	RCal	%Ft	P	F	C	Na
Haddock:										
broiled	4 oz.	0	1	135	119	40	20	6	0	101
fried, breaded	4 oz.	1	1	180	165	35	23	7	6	193
smoked	4 oz.	0	0	120	103	8	26	1	0	90
Halibut	4 oz.	0	1	200	171	41	29	9	0	157
Ham:										
baked	4 oz.	0	3	320	374	69	23	25	0	55
broiled	1 oz.	0	1	75	265	60	5	6	0	13
canned, boneless	4 oz.	0	2	215	193	57	21	14	0	37
Hamburger, see Sandwiches										
Hazelnuts	2 oz.	0	5	380	634	88	8	37	9	1
Headcheese	1 oz.	0	1	75	268	72	4	6	T	332
Herring:										
kippered	1 small	0	2	190	211	62	22	13	0	3,946
pickled	1 small	0	2	215	223	63	20	15	0	3,946
Hickorynuts	2 oz.	0	5	415	673	85	7	39	7	
Honey	1 Tbs.	3	0	65	304	0	T	0	17	1
Honeydew Melon,										
7'' diameter	2'' wedge	0	0	50	33	0	T	0	13	18
Horseradish	1 tsp.	0	0	5	38	3	T	T	1	13
Ice cream	1 scoop	2	1	150	207	54	3	9	15	29
Ice cream cone, cone only	1	1	0	20	377	5	T	T	4	
Ice cream soda	8 oz.	7	1	285	126	28	3	9	50	53
Ice cream sundae	1 avg.	7	3	450	220	50	7	25	50	97
Ice milk	1/2 cup	3	1	180	152	30	5	6	21	89
Ices	1 scoop	5	0	120	78	T	T	T	27	T
Icing, cake, carmel	4 oz.	14	1	408	360	20	1	8	83	94
chocolate	4 oz.	11	2	426	376	38	4	16	66	69
coconut	4 oz.	14	1	412	364	20	2	9	81	133
white	4 oz.	15	1	426	376	15	1	7	90	56
Jams & preserves	1 Tbs.	2	0	55	272	T	T	T	14	3
Jellies	1 Tbs.	2	0	55	273	T	T	T	13	5
Jell-O - see Gelatin										
Jerusalem artichoke	4 oz.	0	0	101	75	1	2	T	20	0
Junket	4 oz.	4	1	150	132	24	3	4	25	56
Kale	4 oz.	0	0	51	53	13	7	T	6	72
Knockwurst	2 oz.	0	2	155	278	75	8	13	T	550
Kohlrabi, boiled	4 oz.	0	0	27	24	4	T	T	6	8
Kumquats, fresh	4 oz.	0	0	75	65	4	1	T	17	8
Lamb chop, broiled	4 oz.	0	3	476	420	79	23	42	0	79
Lamb, roasted leg of	4 oz.	0	3	320	279	56	30	20	0	79
Lamb, shoulder	4 oz.	0	4	390	338	74	25	32	0	79
Lard	1 Tbs.	0	2	125	902	100	0	14	0	0
Leeks	1 piece	0	0	7	52	2	1	T	1	1
Lemon 2'' diameter	1	0	0	20	27	9	T	T	5	1
Lemon juice	1 Tbs.	0	0	5	25	8	T	T	1	T
Lemon peel, candied	1 oz.	4	0	90	316	1	T	T	24	2
Lemonade	1 cup	4	0	100	44	T	T	T	25	1
Lentils, baked	1 cup	0	0	210	41	2	18	T	34	19
Lettuce	2 leaves	0	0	7	13	6	T	T	1	5
Lettuce hearts	4 oz.	0	0	15	13	8	1	T	3	10
Lettuce, romaine	4 oz.	0	0	25	18	15	2	T	4	12
Lichee nuts, dried (Litchi)	1 oz.	0	0	65	229	10	1	T	15	1

Item	Portion	RCU	FU	Cal	RCal	%Ft	P	F	C	Na
Lime, 1 1/2″ diameter	1	0	0	20	28	2	T	T	5	1
Lime juice, fresh	1 cup	0	0	60	26	3	0	T	18	2
Limeade	4 oz.	7	0	210	41	T	T	T	53	T
Liver:										
beef, fried	4 oz.	0	2	260	229	42	30	12	6	209
calves, fried	4 oz.	0	2	290	261	47	33	15	4	134
chicken	4 oz.	0	1	185	165	24	30	5	2	69
Liver paste	2 oz.	0	3	260	462	87	6	25	3	420
Liverwurst	2 oz.	0	2	170	307	79	8	15	2	550
Lobster, baked or broiled	4 oz.	0	1	125	119	36	17	5	T	275
Lobster, newberg	4 oz.	0	1	195	194	51	19	11	3	229
Lobster tails	4 oz.	0	0	100	95	18	21	2	T	221
Loganberries, fresh	1 cup	0	0	90	62	9	T	T	22	1
canned	1 cup	0	0	160	54	9	T	T	40	4
Loquats, flesh only	4 oz.	0	0	54	48	5	T	T	14	0
MSG (Mono Sodium Glutamate)	1 tsp.	0	0	0	0	0	0	0	0	742
Macadamia nuts	2 oz.	0	5	390	691	92	4	40	9	0
Macaroni, cooked	4 oz.	3	0	125	111	3	4	T	39	1
Macaroni & cheese	1 cup	4	3	465	215	46	18	24	43	1,086
Macaroni salad	1 cup	2	3	260	115	69	4	20	26	150
Mackerel, broiled	4 oz.	0	2	265	236	58	25	17	0	120
canned	4 oz.	0	2	190	183	57	21	12	0	240
Mangos	4 oz.	0	0	75	66	6	T	T	19	8
Margarine, regular	1 Tbs.	0	2	100	720	100	T	11	0	137
Blue Bonnet Light	1 Tbs.	0	2	80	576	100	0	9	0	70
Diet Imperial	1 Tbs.	0	1	50	360	100	0	6	0	136
Diet Mazola	1 Tbs.	0	1	50	360	100	0	6	0	144
Parkay Light	1 Tbs.	0	1	70	504	100	0	8	0	120
Marmalade	1 Tbs.	2	0	55	257	T	T	T	14	3
Mayonnaise	1 Tbs.	0	1	90	718	100	T	10	T	75
Meat Loaf	4 oz.	0	2	225	200	60	17	15	3	127
Melon balls	1 cup	0	0	55	26	3	1	T	12	22
Milk:										
buttermilk	1 cup	0	0	85	36	3	9	T	12	307
chocolate flavored	1 cup	2	1	200	85	36	8	8	25	111
dried, skimmed	1 Tbs.	0	0	30	363	2	3	T	3	44
dried, whole	1 Tbs.	0	0	40	502	45	2	2	2	32
Evaporated	1/2 cup	0	1	113	137	32	8	4	11	97
goat's	1/2 cup	0	1	90	67	50	4	5	5	46
malted	1 cup	3	1	235	104	38	9	10	30	206
skimmed, no fat	1 cup	0	0	85	36	3	9	T	13	123
1% fat	1 cup	0	0	100	44	18	8	2	12	130
1% fat w/added milk solids	1 cup	0	0	105	46	17	9	2	12	135
2% fat	1 cup	0	1	120	53	38	8	5	12	140
2% fat w/added milk solids	1 cup	0	1	125	59	36	9	5	12	145
whole milk	1 cup	0	1	170	66	53	9	10	8	131
Lucern, 1/2% fat, Safeway	1 cup	0	0	90	40	10	9	1	12	130
Lucern, 2-10, Safeway	1 cup	0	1	140	62	32	10	5	13	145
Milk Shake										
Burger King, Vanilla	1	7	1	340		29	8	11	52	320
McDonald's, Chocolate	1	8	1	364		22	11	9	60	329
Wendy's Frosty	1	7	2	390		37	9	16	54	247

Item	Portion	RCU	FU	Cal	RCal	%Ft	P	F	C	Na
Molasses	1/4 cup	9	0	207	364	T	0	T	52	12
Muffins, 3'' diameter (most)	1	1	1	120	294	30	3	4	17	180
Mushrooms, raw	4 oz.	0	0	35	28	9	3	T	5	19
broiled with butter	4 oz.	0	1	65	57	69	2	5	3	923
canned	1 cup	0	0	40	17	5	5	T	6	941
Mustard	1 Tbs.	0	0	10	75	53	T	T	T	167
Mustard greens	1 cup	0	0	30	31	16	3	T	5	30
Napoleon pastry	1	3	2	300	464	45	7	15	30	368
Nectarines	1	0	0	40	64	T	1	T	12	4
Noodles, egg, cooked	1 cup	3	0	200	125	9	7	2	37	3
Noodles, chow mein, canned	1 cup	2	1	211	489	47	5	11	23	
Noodle-Roni, mix	4 oz.	2	1	155	137	29	2	5	25	250
Ocean Perch, breaded, fried	3 oz.	1	1	195	229	51	16	11	6	175
Oils, all	1 Tbs.	0	2	125	884	100	0	14	0	0
Oils, all	1/4 cup	0	9	487	884	100	0	54	0	0
Okra, raw	1 cup	0	0	50	36	8	3	T	10	4
cooked	1 cup	0	0	46	29	10	3	T	9	4
Olives, green	4 med.	0	0	15	129	98	T	2	T	310
Olives, ripe	2 large	0	0	15	338	96	T	2	T	95
Omelet	2 egg	0	2	150	173	72	11	12	T	223
Onion, mature, raw	1 avg.	0	0	40	38	3	2	T	10	11
cooked	1 cup	0	0	60	29	3	3	T	14	14
Onion, green	6	0	0	20	45	5	1	T	4	2
Onions, creamed	1/2 cup	0	1	65	57	55	3	4	8	330
Onion rings, french fried	2 oz.	1	2	168	296	80	2	15	17	415
Orange	1 med.	0	0	70	49	4	1	T	17	1
Orange juice:										
canned or frozen, diluted	1 cup	0	0	120	45	4	2	T	28	3
fresh	1 cup	0	0	110	45	4	2	1	26	2
frozen concentrate	6 oz.	3	0	360	158	5	5	T	87	5
Orange-apricot juice	1 cup	0	0	125	50	2	1	T	32	T
Orange-grapefruit juice	1 cup	0	0	110	49	T	1	T	26	2
Orange-pineapple drink	1 cup	1	0	120	53	T	T	T	29	1
Orange peel, candied	2 oz.	4	0	190	316	1	T	T	48	
Ovaltine with skim milk	1 cup	0	0	160	71	6	11	1	22	219
with whole milk	1 cup	0	1	240	106	38	11	10	22	227
Oysters:										
canned	4 oz.	0	0	86	76	10	10	1	6	250
fried	4 oz.	0	2	270	239	53	10	16	21	233
raw	1 cup	0	1	160	91	23	20	4	8	177
Pancake, 4'' diameter	1	1	0	60	231	30	2	2	9	110
with butter & syrup	3	3	5	450	578	64	6	32	30	496
Papaya, raw	1 cup	0	0	70	39	2	1	T	18	5
Parsley, fresh	1 Tbs.	0	0	1	44	15	T	T	T	1
Parsnips, cooked	1 cup	0	0	100	66	7	2	1	23	12
Passion fruit	4 oz.	0	0	102	90	6	T	T	24	32
Pate de fois gras	1 Tbs.	0	1	85	462	85	2	8	1	105
Peaches:										
canned in heavy syrup	1 cup	5	0	200	78	1	1	T	52	5
canned in water	1 cup	0	0	75	31	3	1	T	20	5
dried, uncooked	1 cup	2	0	420	262	2	5	1	99	26
dried, cooked, unsweetened	1 cup	1	0	220	82	1	3	1	58	13
raw, sliced	1 cup	0	0	65	38	2	1	T	16	2

Item	Portion	RCU	FU	Cal	RCal	%Ft	P	F	C	Na
raw, whole, 2'' diameter	1 cup	0	0	38	38	2	T	T	10	1
Peanut butter	1 Tbs.	0	1	95	582	76	4	8	3	98
Peanuts, roasted & salted	1/2 cup	0	8	760	585	77	33	65	14	780
Pears, raw, 3'' long	1	0	0	100	61	5	1	T	25	3
Pears, canned	1 cup	5	0	195	76	2	1	1	47	3
Pear juice nectar	1 cup	0	0	100	52	4	T	T	24	1
Peas, green, canned	1/2 cup	0	0	75	88	4	4	T	14	268
fresh, cooked	1/2 cup	0	0	55	71	5	3	T	10	1
Peas, dried, cooked	4 oz.	0	0	85	115	2	6	T	14	10
Peas, black-eyed, canned	4 oz.	0	0	85	70	2	6	T	14	33
Pecans, halves	1 cup	0	9	740	687	85	10	70	16	T
chopped	1 Tbs.	0	1	50	687	90	T	5	1	T
Peppers, green fresh	1 med.	0	0	13	22	8	T	T	3	8
Peppers, hot green	4 oz.	0	0	31	37	4	T	T	8	12
Pepper, hot red	4 oz.	0	0	54	65	26	2	2	8	21
Persimmons	1 avg.	0	0	100	127	3	1	T	24	8
Pickles:										
cucumber	4 spears	0	0	25	73	2	1	T	5	230
dill or sour	1 large	0	0	10	11	16	T	T	3	1,298
sweet	1 small	0	0	20	146	2	T	T	5	119
Pickle relish	1 Tbs.	2	0	12	19	4	T	T	24	62
Pies:										
apple or cherry	4'' wedge	7	2	350	256	39	3	15	50	411
blackberry	4'' wedge	5	2	275	243	39	3	12	38	303
butterscotch	4'' wedge	6	2	350	267	36	6	14	50	281
custard	4'' wedge	4	2	285	218	44	8	14	30	375
lemon meringue	4'' wedge	6	2	305	255	35	4	12	45	337
mince	4'' wedge	7	2	365	271	39	3	16	56	603
pecan	4'' wedge	8	3	490	418	50	6	27	60	259
pumpkin	4'' wedge	4	2	275	211	49	5	15	32	279
strawberry	4'' wedge	7	1	340	198	24	2	9	56	333
Pie crust	1 shell	7	8	900	500	60	11	60	79	1,100
Pig's feet, pickled	4 oz.	0	2	225	199	64	18	16	T	1,000
Pimientos, canned	4 oz.	0	0	30	27	17	1	T	6	42
Pineapple:										
canned in heavy syrup	1 slice	1	0	50	74	2	T	T	12	1
canned in low calorie syrup	1/2 cup	0	0	45	39	2	T	T	11	1
fresh	1 cup	0	0	75	52	2	1	T	19	2
Pineapple juice	1 cup	0	0	135	55	1	1	T	34	2
Pine nuts	2 oz.	0	3	310	635	78	17	27	7	180
Pistachio nuts	16	0	1	50	594	90	2	5	2	32
Pizza, cheese	6'' wedge	2	1	185	236	29	7	6	27	550
Pizza Hut, Thin'n Crispy 13''	1/2	4	1	340		29	19	11	42	900
Pizza Hut, Thick'n Chewy 10''	1/2	4	2	450		32	25	16	52	900
Plums, fresh, 2'' diameter	1	0	0	25	66	2	T	T	7	1
canned	1 cup	4	0	205	63	1	1	T	53	9
Pomegranate, raw, whole	1 pound	0	0	160	63	4	T	T	40	8
Popcorn, popped, plain	1 cup	0	0	55	386	16	2	1	11	T
with butter and salt	1 cup	0	2	155	456	70	2	12	11	659
Popovers	1	1	0	75	112	36	3	3	11	74

Item	Portion	RCU	FU	Cal	RCal	%Ft	P	F	C	Na
Pork:										
Boston butt cured	4 oz.	0	3	320	251	76	17	27	0	78
chops, baked or broiled	1 med.	0	2	275	373	52	30	16	0	50
chops, fried	1 med.	0	3	375	508	65	30	27	0	63
Roast, lean	3 oz.	0	1	196	230	51	24	11	0	55
Potato chips	10 chips	0	1	115	568	63	1	8	10	200
Potatoes, white:										
baked	1 med.	0	0	90	93	1	3	T	21	4
boiled	1 med.	0	0	80	76	1	2	T	18	3
french fried	10 pieces	0	1	155	274	41	2	7	20	133
Burger King	1 serving	0	1	210		47	3	11	25	230
Skipper's	1 serving	0	3	388		51	6	22	46	250
Wendy's	1 serving	0	2	330		44	5	16	41	240
mashed with milk	1 cup	0	0	125	65	7	4	1	25	579
Potatoes, sweet - see sweet potatoes										
Pretzels, thin, twisted	2	1	0	46	383	12	1	1	9	202
stick, 2 1/2" long	20	0	0	23	390	8	1	T	4	48
Protein supplements:										
Bronson Super Protein, Vanilla	1 oz.	1	0	110	388	8	16	1	9	T
with 8 oz. skim milk	1 oz.	1	0	200	78	5	25	1	21	124
Carnation Slender	1 pkg.	2	0	104	366	4	10	T	16	170
Soup-R-Fast, Robard	1 pkg.	0	0	60	26	0	15	0	0	T
Prune Juice	4 oz.	0	0	95	77	1	1	T	23	2
Prunes:										
cooked with sugar	4 oz.	2	0	205	180	1	1	T	50	5
dried	4	0	0	100	255	2	1	T	24	3
stewed without sugar	4 oz.	0	0	165	119	2	1	T	40	6
Pudding:										
bread	1/2 cup	4	1	210	187	30	6	7	32	279
butterscotch	1/2 cup	4	1	140	110	19	3	3	23	250
chocolate	1/2 cup	5	1	193	148	30	4	6	34	73
rice	1/2 cup	3	0	165	146	16	4	3	30	94
tapioca	1/2 cup	2	1	110	134	33	4	4	14	128
vanilla	1/2 cup	2	1	143	111	31	5	5	20	84
Pumpkin, canned	1 cup	0	0	80	33	11	2	1	18	5
Pumpkin seeds	1 oz.	0	2	155	553	75	8	13	4	T
Quail, broiled	4 oz.	0	1	190	168	38	28	8	0	44
Quince, fresh	1	0	0	50	57	2	T	T	12	4
Quinine water	6 oz.	2	0	50	29	0	0	0	12	10
Rabbit	4 oz.	0	1	240	216	41	34	11	0	46
Radishes	4 small	0	0	8	17	5	T	T	2	8
Raisins	1/2 cup	2	0	240	289	1	2	T	58	22
Raspberries, black, fresh	1 cup	0	0	80	73	23	2	2	16	1
Raspberries, red, fresh	1 cup	0	0	70	57	13	3	1	17	1
Red snapper, raw	4 oz.	0	0	100	93	9	22	1	0	72
Rhubarb, raw, diced	1 cup	0	0	18	16	6	1	T	5	2
cooked with sugar	1 cup	15	0	385	141	1	1	T	98	5
Rice, brown, cooked (MJB)	1/2 cup	0	0	78	87	11	2	1	17	357
cooked white	1/2 cup	0	0	112	109	1	2	T	25	270
instant white, cooked	1/2 cup	0	0	90	128	T	2	T	25	1
raw white	1/2 cup	0	0	335	363	1	6	T	75	5

Item	Portion	RCU	FU	Cal	RCal	%Ft	P	F	C	Na
Rice, wild, raw	1/2 cup	0	0	400	361	2	16	1	85	6
cooked	1/2 cup	0	0	85	75	11	3	1	15	201
Rice-A-Roni	4 oz.	0	1	175	154	26	2	5	30	400
Rutabaga, boiled	1/2 cup	0	0	40	35	3	1	T	9	5
Salad dressing:										
Bleu cheese	1 Tbs.	0	1	75	504	84	T	7	2	164
French	1 Tbs.	0	1	66	410	82	T	6	3	105
Italian	1 Tbs.	0	1	83	552	87	T	8	1	314
Mayonnaise	1 Tbs.	0	2	90	718	99	T	10	T	88
Roquefort	1 Tbs.	0	1	76	504	95	1	8	T	164
Russian	1 Tbs.	0	1	74	494	97	T	8	T	130
Thousand Island	1 Tbs.	0	1	70	502	90	T	7	2	112
Salad dressing, low calorie:										
Bleu cheese, Kraft	1 Tbs.	0	0	13	76	69	1	1	T	286
Catalina, Kraft	1 Tbs.	0	0	15	100	60	T	1	1	110
French, Kraft	1 Tbs.	0	0	21	156	86	T	2	1	267
Imitation Mayonnaise	1 Tbs.	0	0	22	155	82	T	2	1	190
Italian, Kraft	1 Tbs.	0	0	10	50	90	T	1	T	173
Russian, Wishbone	1 Tbs.	0	0	24	170	38	T	1	3	162
Thousand Island, Kraft	1 Tbs.	0	0	28	180	64	T	2	2	133
Salad dressing from Good										
Seasons mix:										
Bleu cheese	1 Tbs.	0	1	89	624	91	T	9	2	170
Thick, Creamy	1 Tbs.	0	1	96	678	84	T	9	4	106
Cheese Garlic	1 Tbs.	0	1	84	594	96	T	9	1	166
French, Old Fashion	1 Tbs.	0	1	83	587	98	T	9	T	270
Thick, Creamy	1 Tbs.	0	1	97	686	84	T	9	4	203
Garlic	1 Tbs.	0	1	84	594	96	T	9	1	166
Italian	1 Tbs.	0	1	84	594	96	T	9	1	166
Thick, Creamy	1 Tbs.	0	1	94	664	86	T	9	3	183
Low Cal	1 Tbs.	0	0	9	64	10	T	T	2	165
Thousand Island	1 Tbs.	0	1	80	565	90	T	8	2	98
Salami	1 oz.	0	1	120	450	83	7	11	T	425
Salt	1 tsp.	0	0	0	0	0	0	0	0	1,890
Salmon, raw	4 oz.	0	2	250	217	68	19	19	0	51
canned	4 oz.	0	2	220	210	61	21	15	0	505
Sandwiches:										
bacon, lettuce & tomato	1	3	4	477	495	62	13	33	32	681
bologna	1	2	3	364	256	59	10	24	27	832
cheeseburger	1	2	5	540	271	62	28	37	22	1,010
chicken salad	1	2	3	334	391	59	10	21	26	529
Club, Arby's	1	4	4	560		48	30	30	43	1,610
egg, fried	1	2	2	322	377	53	11	19	27	474
egg, salad with mayonnaise	1	2	2	355	415	41	24	16	29	488
Egg McMuffin, McDonald's	1	2	3	352		51	18	20	26	914
Fillet-O-Fish, McDonald's	1	3	3	402		51	15	23	34	709
ham salad	1	2	3	345	404	57	11	22	26	371
ham, sliced	1	2	2	265	200	41	11	12	28	357
ham, with swiss cheese	1	2	3	370	296	49	18	20	29	558
Ham'n Cheese, Arby's	1	3	2	380		40	23	17	33	1,350
hamburger	1	2	4	435	255	58	22	28	21	550
Burger King Whopper	1	4	5	630		51	26	36	50	990
McDonald's Big Mac	1	3	4	541		52	26	31	39	962

Item	Portion	RCU	FU	Cal	RCal	%Ft	P	F	C	Na
Wendy's Single	1	3	3	470		50	26	26	34	774
with cheese	1	3	4	580		53	33	34	34	1,085
Wendy's Double	1	3	5	670		54	44	40	34	980
with cheese	1	3	6	800		54	50	48	41	1,414
Wendy's Triple	1	3	6	850		54	65	51	33	1,217
with cheese	1	3	9	1040		59	72	68	35	1,848
roast beef	1	2	1	365	427	27	39	11	24	870
Jr. Roast Beef, Arby's	1	2	1	220		41	12	10	21	530
Roast Beef, Arby's	1	3	2	350		39	22	15	32	880
with cheese	1	3	3	450		44	27	22	36	1,220
Super Roast Beef, Arby's	1	5	4	620		41	30	28	61	1,420
tomato and lettuce	1	3	3	344	202	58	6	22	31	464
tuna salad (oil pack tuna)	1	2	3	390	456	48	22	21	28	707
turkey	1	3	1	325	228	22	25	8	38	329
Turkey Delux, Arby's	1	4	3	510		42	28	24	46	1,220
Sardines, canned	4 oz.	0	2	230	196	47	29	12	1	932
Sauce:										
barbecue	1 Tbs.	0	1	50	567	90	2	5	T	130
chili	1 Tbs.	0	0	17	359	41	0	T	4	201
soy	1 Tbs.	0	0	12	253	29	T	T	3	1,293
tarter	1 Tbs.	0	1	75	850	96	T	8	T	90
tomato	1 cup	2	0	75	33	4	T	T	19	1,252
white, medium	1 Tbs.	0	0	25	528	72	1	2	1	60
Worcestershire	1 Tbs.	0	0	10	211	11	T	T	2	175
Sauerkraut	1/2 cup	0	0	25	93	11	1	T	5	1,037
Sausage: canned pork	4 oz.	0	5	425	381	87	21	37	2	1,784
Polish	4 oz.	0	4	340	304	77	18	29	1	884
pork, 3" x 1 1/4" dia. link	1	0	4	339	497	93	6	35	T	503
4" x 1 1/4" dia. link 1 oz.	1	0	3	141	497	93	3	14	T	210
Vienna, canned	4 oz.	0	3	540	240	75	31	45	1	1,693
Scallions	5	0	0	20		T	1	T	5	1
Scallops, broiled	4 oz.	0	0	140	112	13	27	2	2	331
fried	4 large	1	1	230	194	35	20	9	15	400
Skipper's	1 serving	2	1	273		30	18	9	29	310
Scrapple	4 oz.	1	2	275	215	37	10	15	26	1,740
Sesame seeds	1 oz.	0	2	165	563	76	5	14	6	18
Shad, baked	4 oz.	0	2	225	201	52	26	13	0	88
Sherbets	1 scoop	5	0	130	134	7	1	1	29	10
Shortening	1 Tbs.	0	2	125	884	100	0	14	0	0
Shrimp:										
broiled	4 oz.	0	0	90	79	10	20	1	2	139
canned	3 oz.	0	0	100	116	9	21	1	T	321
French fried	10 avg.	1	2	240	225	45	23	12	11	198
fried	3 jumbo	0	1	100	345	36	8	4	8	85
Skipper's	1 serving	2	2	278		42	14	13	27	230
Shrimp cocktail	6 med.	0	0	75	324	12	16	1	1	2
Soft Drinks, diet:										
Canada Dry Sugar Free	12 oz.	0	0	1	0	0	0	0	T	17
Diet Pepsi-Cola or Light	12 oz.	0	0	1	0	0	0	0	T	62
Diet Rite, Sugar Free	12 oz.	0	0	1	0	0	0	0	T	58
Diet Shasta	12 oz.	0	0	1	0	0	0	0	T	74
Fresca	12 oz.	0	0	4	1	0	0	0	1	62
R C Cola, sugar free	12 oz.	0	0	1	0	0	0	0	T	58

Item	Portion	RCU	FU	Cal	RCal	%Ft	P	F	C	Na
R C 100	12 oz.	0	0	1	0	0	0	0	T	58
Tab	12 oz.	0	0	1	0	0	0	0	T	26
Soft Drinks, regular:										
Coke:										
Coca Cola	12 oz.	7	0	144	42	0	0	0	36	T
Pepsi-Cola	12 oz.	7	0	157	46	0	0	0	39	T
Shasta	12 oz.	7	0	143	42	0	0	0	36	T
R C	12 oz.	7	0	151	44	0	0	0	38	T
Ginger Ale:										
Fanta	12 oz.	7	0	126	37	0	0	0	32	T
Shasta	12 oz.	7	0	117	34	0	0	0	29	T
Dr. Pepper	12 oz.	7	0	149	44	0	0	0	37	T
Mountain Dew	12 oz.	7	0	178	52	0	0	0	45	T
Mr. Pibb	12 oz.	7	0	140	41	0	0	0	35	T
Orange:										
Fanta	12 oz.	7	0	176	52	0	0	0	44	T
Shasta	12 oz.	7	0	143	42	0	0	0	36	T
Root Beer:										
Fanta	12 oz.	7	0	155	46	0	0	0	19	T
Hires	12 oz.	7	0	166	49	0	0	0	42	T
Shasta	12 oz.	7	0	150	44	0	0	0	38	T
Most other flavors	12 oz.	7	0	150	44	0	0	0	38	T
Sole, fillet, broiled	4 oz.	0	0	90	79	11	20	T	0	88
fried	4 oz.	0	1	125	110	36	20	5	0	190
Soup:										
bean	1 cup	0	1	170	67	32	8	6	22	1,023
beef broth	1 cup	0	0	30	13	20	5	1	3	752
chicken noodle	1 cup	0	0	55	26	33	3	2	6	863
chicken, cream of	1 cup	0	1	90	39	60	2	6	8	932
chicken with rice	1 cup	0	0	45	20	20	2	1	6	860
clam chowder,										
New England	1 cup	0	1	95	42	57	2	6	6	766
Manhattan	1 cup	0	0	60	33	30	2	2	8	696
lentil	1 cup	0	0	180	79	10	4	2	40	566
minestrone	1 cup	0	0	105	32	26	5	3	14	991
mushroom, cream of	1 cup	0	2	215	56	59	7	14	16	1,528
oyster stew	1 cup	0	1	150	66	30	5	5	21	524
potato, cream of	1 cup	0	1	200	88	45	8	10	16	1,049
split pea	1 cup	0	0	145	64	19	9	3	21	1,004
tomato	1 cup	0	0	90	36	30	2	3	16	990
tomato, cream of	1 cup	0	1	175	69	36	7	7	23	1,070
turkey	1 cup	0	0	70	33	13	2	1	13	882
vegetable	1 cup	0	0	80	32	23	5	2	10	885
Soy beans, cooked	1 cup	0	2	234	118	40	20	10	19	536
dried	1/2 cup	0	2	123	404	40	36	19	35	249
Soy bean curd (2x3x1 in.)	1 piece	0	0	89	72	53	10	5	3	8
Spaghetti, cooked	1 cup	3	0	155	111	6	5	1	32	1
with meat ball and										
tomato sauce	1 cup	3	2	330	134	33	19	12	39	1,002
with tomato sauce & cheese	1 cup	3	1	260	104	31	9	9	37	995
Spaghetti sauce, with meat	1 cup	1	1	220	97	33	6	8	31	1,508
without meat	1 cup	1	1	220	97	33	4	8	32	1,540

Item	Portion	RCU	FU	Cal	RCal	%Ft	P	F	C	Na
Spinach:										
canned	1 cup	0	0	45	24	20	5	1	6	443
cooked, fresh	1 cup	0	0	40	23	23	5	1	5	86
raw	1/2 pound	0	0	60	26	15	7	1	6	164
Squab, broiled	1/2 med.	0	1	160		45	20	8	0	100
roasted	1/2 med.	0	1	190		52	23	11	0	120
Squash, cooked summer	1 cup	0	0	30	14	7	2	T	7	2
cooked winter	1 cup	0	0	130	63	6	4	1	32	2
Stew:										
beef & vegetable	1 cup	0	1	200	88	45	14	10	14	91
chicken	1 cup	0	1	166	73	33	12	6	16	1,018
Irish or lamb	1 cup	0	3	470	207	50	30	26	30	910
Strawberries, raw	1 cup	0	0	55	37	12	1	1	12	1
frozen and sweetened	1 cup	7	0	250	109	2	2	T	54	2
Sturgeon, smoked	2 oz.	0	0	70	149	13	17	1	0	140
Succotash	1/2 cup	0	0	110	93	4	5	T	21	45
Sugar, granulated	1 Tbs.	2	0	46	385	0	0	0	12	T
Sugar, granulated	1/2 cup	17	0	385	385	0	0	0	88	T
Sugar, brown, packed	1/2 cup	9	0	206	373	0	0	0	53	33
Sugar, powdered	1 cup	10	0	231	385	0	0	0	60	1
Sunflower seeds, hulled	1 oz.	0	2	159	560	68	7	12	6	9
Sweet potatoes:										
baked	1 med.	0	0	155	141	6	2	1	36	13
boiled	1 med.	0	0	170	114	5	2	1	39	15
candied	4 oz.	4	1	197	168	18	1	4	40	49
canned	1 cup	0	0	235	114	2	4	T	54	99
Swordfish, broiled	4 oz.	0	1	200	174	36	31	8	0	140
Syrups:										
caramel	1 Tbs.	3	0	65	459	0	0	0	16	T
chocolate, thin type	1 Tbs.	1	0	35	247	6	T	T	8	10
corn	1 Tbs.	2	0	50	352	2	T	T	12	14
maple	1 Tbs.	2	0	50	352	0	0	0	13	2
molasses, blackstrap	1 Tbs.	2	0	45	317	1	T	T	11	18
molasses, medium	1 Tbs.	2	0	50	352	T	T	T	13	7
sorghum	1 Tbs.	2	0	55	388	T	T	T	14	13
Taco Bell Taco	1	0	1	185		39	15	8	14	79
Taco Time:										
Burrito, meat	1	2	2	291		43	20	14	23	848
Burrito, soft bean	1	2	2	314		37	13	13	37	762
Taco	1-	0	1	195		42	14	9	14	591
Soft Flour Taco	1	1	2	295		43	19	20	24	686
Supreme	1	1	3	356		51	19	20	24	696
Tangerine	1 med.	0	0	40	46	4	1	T	10	2
Tangerine juice, canned	1 cup	0	0	125	43	7	1	1	30	3
Tea	1 cup	0	0	2	2	T	T	T	T	T
Thuringer Salami	1 oz.	0	1	87	307	8	4	8	T	292
Toast:										
cinnamon &										
sugar,　white bread	1 slice	4	1	200	414	27	7	6	29	117
French with 1 Tbs. syrup	1 piece	3	0	150		24	4	4	23	220
Melba	1 slice	1	0	30		T	1	T	4	35
Tomato aspic	1/2 cup	0	0	60		T	T	T	14	141
Tomato juice	1 cup	0	0	45	19	5	2	T	10	474

Item	Portion	RCU	FU	Cal	RCal	%Ft	P	F	C	Na
Tomato paste, canned	6 oz.	0	0	140	82	4	6	T	31	65
Tomato puree, canned	4 oz.	0	0	50	39	4	2	T	9	512
Tomatoes, canned or stewed	1 cup	0	0	50	21	9	2	1	10	310
Tomatoes, fresh	1 med.	0	0	40	22	8	2	T	9	5
Tongue, beef, boiled	4 oz.	0	2	280	244	62	25	19	1	69
Tongue, pickled	4 oz.	0	3	307	270	67	23	23	1	500
Toppings:										
butterscotch	1 Tbs.	3	0	63	444	5	T	T	15	35
caramel	1 Tbs.	3	0	61	430	4	T	T	15	55
chocolate, thin type	1 Tbs.	2	0	45	317	2	T	T	12	10
chocolate fudge	1 Tbs.	2	0	63	444	29	1	2	10	9
Cool Whip	1 Tbs.	0	0	16	113	56	T	1	1	1
Dream Whip	1 Tbs.	0	0	14	99	T	T	T	2	4
marshmallow creme	1 Tbs.	2	0	45	317	T	T	T	12	9
pineapple or strawberry	1 Tbs.	2	0	40	282	T	T	T	10	1
Tortilla, corn	1	0	0	55		16	1	1	10	158
Tortilla, flour	1	3	1	214		29	5	7	32	192
Tripe pickled	4 oz.	0	0	60	62	15	13	1	0	52
Trout, fried	1 avg.	0	3	350		69	24	27	T	80
Tuna, canned in oil, drained	3 1/4 oz.	0	1	184	197	39	27	8	0	511
Breast of Chicken, w/liquid	3 1/4 oz.	0	3	270	288	67	22	0	0	536
Chicken of the Sea,										
w/liquid	3 1/4 oz.	0	2	203	217	58	22	13	0	598
Light Chunk, drained	3 1/4 oz.	0	1	147	157	43	22	7	0	536
Del Monte Light Chunk	3 1/4 oz.	0	2	239	286	64	22	17	0	575
Tuna, canned in water:										
Chicken of the Sea, light	3 1/4 oz.	0	0	112	120	16	24	2	0	553
solid white, drained	3 1/4 oz.	0	0	108	127	8	25	1	0	553
Dietetic drained	3 1/4 oz.	0	0	100	107	9	22	1	0	37
Turkey:										
roasted	4 oz.	0	1	250	223	40	35	11	0	171
all dark meat	4 oz.	0	1	230	203	35	33	9	0	121
all white meat	4 oz.	0	0	200	176	18	37	4	0	93
Turnip greens, cooked	1 cup	0	0	45	20	9	4	T	8	45
Turnips, cooked	1 cup	0	0	50	23	8	2	T	10	74
Turnovers, fruit	1 med.	4	1	250		36	3	10	37	251
V-8 Juice	1 cup	0	0	45	19	5	2	T	9	872
low sodium	1 cup	0	0	45	19	5	2	T	9	60
Veal:										
chop	1 med.	0	2	260	181	52	30	15	0	97
cutlet, breaded	4 oz.	1	1	230	154	43	24	11	8	87
roast	4 oz.	0	2	245	164	70	31	19	0	91
steak	4 oz.	0	2	265	173	51	40	15	0	98
stew	4 oz.	0	2	235	207	50	15	13	15	200
Venison, raw, lean	4 oz.	0	1	143	126	44	20	7	0	60
Vermicelli, cooked	1 cup	3	0	155	70	6	5	1	32	1
Vinegar	2 Tbs.	0	0	5	12	T	T	T	1	T
Vienna sausage	2	0	1	76	240	74	5	6	T	126
Waffles, plain	1 med.	2	2	225	279	48	10	12	28	561
Walnuts	10	0	4	355	651	71	11	28	8	1
Water, tap	1 cup	0	0	0	0	0	0	0	0	2
artifically softened	1 cup	0	0	0	0	0	0	0	0	147

Item	Portion	RCU	FU	Cal	RCal	%Ft	P	F	C	Na
Perrier Water	1 cup	0	0	0	0	0	0	0	0	4
Vichy water	1 cup	0	0	0	0	0	0	0	0	331
Watercress, raw	4 oz.	0	0	25	19	15	2	T	4	68
Watermelon, 3/4" x 10" diameter	1 slice	0	0	84	26	11	2	1	17	4
Welsh rarebit	1 cup	2	4	430	179	63	18	30	22	798
Wheat bran, miller's, fine	1 Tbs.	0	0	19	213	11	2	T	3	1
regular flakes	1 Tbs.	0	0	14	213	11	1	T	2	1
Wheat germ	1 Tbs.	0	0	55	363	16	4	1	7	1
Whitefish, baked	4 oz.	0	2	210	215	69	17	16	0	246
smoked	4 oz.	0	1	175	155	41	23	8	0	205
Wine:										
Cooking sherry	4 oz.	2	0	38	34	0	0	0	10	660
Dessert (18.8% alcohol)	4 oz.	7	0	163	138	0	0	0	41	5
Table (12.2% alcohol)	4 oz.	4	0	100	85	0	0	0	25	5
Wienerschnitzel	7 oz.	1	3	480	241	39	25	21	7	240
Yeast, bakers, dry	1 oz.	0	0	85	282	6	10	T	3	16
Yeast, brewers, dry	1 Tbs.	0	0	50	283	3	5	T	3	21
Yogurt, skimmed milk	1 cup	0	0	125	50	31	8	4	13	128
made with whole milk	1 cup	0	1	150	62	50	7	8	12	114
Skim milk with fruit	1 cup	4	0	250	100	13	8	4	46	130

Daily Record

Date _____

Time	Amount	Item	RCU	FU	D U	H
se		Water	Total			

Time	Amount	Item	RCU	FU	D U	H
:ise		Water	Total			

Meal: **B** = breakfast, **L** = light meal, **M** = main meal, **S** = snack.
H = hunger. Put an X for no hunger prior to snack

End of Main Meal Hunger/Satiety	**Points**
Completely satisfied	10
No hunger, but not completely satisfied	8
Slightly overfull or mild hunger	5
Definately overfull or moderate hunger	0

PROGRESS SUMMARY

Month	Day
EXERCISE	**Poss**
First 30 min. (½ pt./min.)	15
31 to 60 min. (1 pt./min.)	30
Correct Rate	5
Subtotal	50
FOOD & DRINK CHOICES	
1. Refined Carbohydrates	10
2. Fat Intake	10
3. Water Drinking	5
Subtotal	25
EATING BEHAVIOR	
4. End Main Meal Hunger	10
5. Meal Frequency	5
6. No Hunger Snacking	5
7. Faulty Drinking	5
Subtotal	25
TOTAL	100

SCORING TABLES

Food and Drink Choices

1. Refined Carbohydrates: Look up RCU's and allocate points as follows:

Total RCU	Pts.
0-2	10
3-4	8
5-6	6
7-8	4
9-10	2
11 or more	0

2. Fat Intake: Look up FU in table and allocate points as follows:

Ideal Weight		
Under 140 lbs.	Over 140 lbs	Pts.
0-4	0-5	10
5	6	7
6	7	3
7 +	8 +	0

3. Water Drinking:

	Pts.
6 glasses or more	5
5	4
4	3
3	2
2	1

Eating Behavior

4. End Main Meal Hunger

	Pts.
Complete satiety	10
No hunger, not satisfied	8
Slightly overfull or slightly hungry	5
Definitely overfull or def. hungry	0

5. Meal Frequency

	Pts.
3 or more	5
2	3
1	0

6. Times Snacking With No Hunger

	Pts.
0	5
1	4
2	3
3	2
4 or more	1

7. Faulty Drinking: 1 DU for any drink except water or skim milk.

DU	Pts.
0-1	5
2	4
3	2
4 or more	0

Daily Record

Date _____

Day	Meal	Time	Amount	Item	RCU	FU	D U	H
Exercise			Water		Total			

Day	Meal	Time	Amount	Item	RCU	FU	D U	H
Exercise			Water		Total			

Meal:**B** = breakfast, **L** = light meal, **M** = main meal, **S** = snack.
H = hunger. Put an X for no hunger prior to snack

End of Main Meal Hunger/Satiety	Points
Completely satisfied	10
No hunger, but not completely satisfied	8
Slightly overfull or mild hunger	5
Definately overfull or moderate hunger	0

Daily Record

Date _____

Day	Meal	Time	Amount	Item	RCU	FU	DU	H
Exercise			Water	Total				

Day	Meal	Time	Amount	Item	RCU	FU	DU	H
Exercise			Water	Total				

Meal: **B** = breakfast, **L** = light meal, **M** = main meal, **S** = snack.
H = hunger. Put an X for no hunger prior to snack

End of Main Meal Hunger/Satiety	Points
Completely satisfied	10
No hunger, but not completely satisfied	8
Slightly overfull or mild hunger	5
Definately overfull or moderate hunger	0

BOOKS

Bjorntorp, Cairella Howard: Recent Advances in Obesity Research: III Proceedings of the 3rd International Congress on Obesity, John Libbey, London, 1980.

Bray, George A.: Comparative Methods of Weight Loss.

Bray, George A.: Obesity in Perspective, Proceedings of the Conference Sponsored by the John E. Fogarty International Center. DHEW Publication Mo. (NIH) 75-708, 1973.

Bray, George A.: Recent Advances in Obesity Research: II Proceedings of the 2nd International Congress on Obesity, Technomic Publishing Company, Inc., 1977.

Bray, George A.: The Obese Patient, W. B. Saunders Company, 1976.

Briggs, G. M. and Calloway, D. H.: Bogert's Nutrition and Physical Fitness, W. B. Saunders Company, 1979.

Chernin, Kim: The Obsession, Harper & Row, 1981.

Deutsch, Ronald M.: Realities of Nutrition, Rule Publishing, 1976.

Edwards, Sandra: Too Much Is Not Enough, McGraw Hill, 1981.

Enzi, G. et al.: Obesity: Pathogenesis and Treatment, Academic Press, 1981.

Fisher, A. Garth and Conlee, Robert K.: The Complete Book of Physical Fitness, BYU Press, 1979.

Halpern, Seymour L.: Quick Reference to Clinical Nutrition, J. B. Lippincott Company, 1979.

Howard, Alan: Recent Advances In Obesity Research: I Proceedings of the 1st International Congress on Obesity, Technomic Publishing Company, Inc., 1974.

Irvine, W. J.: Clinics In Endrocrinology and Metabolism, W. B. Saunders Company, 1975.

Orbach, Susie: Fat Is A Feminist Issue, Berkley, 1978.

Schneider, Howard A. et al.: Nutritional Support of Medical Practice, Harper & Row, 1977.

Stuart, R. B. and Davis, B.: Slim Chance In A Fat World, Research Press Co., 1972.

Stunkard, Albert J.: Obesity, W. B. Saunders Company, 1980.

Stunkard, Albert J.: The Pain of Obesity, Bull Publishing, 1976.

U.S. Dept. of Agriculture: Nutritive Value of American Foods, Agriculture Handbook No. 456, 1975.

U.S. Dept. of Agriculture: Composition of Foods, Agriculture Handbook No. 8, 1963.

Wolman, B. B.: Psychological Aspects of Obesity, Van Nostrand Reinhold, 1982.

ARTICLES - Regulation of Body Weight

Ahlskog, J.E., and Hoebel, B. G.: Overeating and obesity from damage to a noradrenergic system in the brain. Science, 182:166-167, 1973.

Antelman, S.M., and Schechtman, H.: Tail pinch induces eating in sated rats which appears to depend on nigrostriatal dopamine. Science, 189:731-733, 1975.

Apfelbaum, M.: Influence of level of energy intake on energy expenditure in man: Effects of spontaneous intake, experimental starvation, and experimental overeating. In Bray, G. A., ed.: Obesity In Perspective. Washington, D.C., U.S. Gov't. Printing Office, 1973.

Barboriak. J.J., Krehl, W. A., Cowgill, G. R., et al.: Influence of high-fat diets on growth and development of obesity in the albino rat. J. Nutr. 69:241-249, 1958.

Blundell, J. E., and Latham, C. J.: Pharmacological manipulation of feeding: possible influences of serotonin and dopamine on food intake. In Samanin, R., and Garattini, S., eds.: Central Mechanisms of Anorectic Drugs. New York, Raven Press, pp. 83-109, 1978.

Blundell, J. E., and Latham, C. J.: Pharmacology of food and water intake. In Cooper, S., and Brown, K., eds: Chemical Influences on Behaviour, London, Academic Press, pp. 201-253, 1979.

Blundell, J.E., and Latham, C. F.: Serotonergic influences on food intake: effect of 5-hydroxytryptophan on parameters of feeding behaviour in deprived and free-feeding rats. Pharm. Biochem. Behav., 11:431-437, 1979.

Blundell, J. E.: Hunger and satiety in the control of food intake: implications for the treatment of obesity. La Clinica Dietologica, 4:3-23, 1977.

Blundell, J. E.: Serotonin and Feeding. In Essman, W. B., and Valzelli, L., eds.: Serotonin in Health and Disease. New York, Spectrum, 1979.

Blundell, J. E.: Hunger, appetite and satiety - constructs in search of identities. In Turner, M.R., ed.: Lifestyles in Nutrition. Cambridge. Cambridge Univ. Press, 1979.

Booth, D.A., and Mather, P.: Prototype model of human feeding, growth and obesity. In Booth, D. A., ed.: Hunger Models: Computable Theory of Feeding Control. London, Academic Press, 1978.

Braun, T., Kazdova, L., Fabry, P., et al.: Meal eating and refeeding after a single fast as a stimulus for increasing the number of fat cells in abdominal adipose tissue of rats. Metab. Clin. Exper., 17:825-832, 1968.

Bray, G. A., and Gallagher, T. F., Jr.: Manifestations of hypothalamic obesity in man: a comprehensive investigation of eight patients and a review of the literature. Medicine, 54:301-330, 1975.

Brooks, C. McC., and Lambert, E. F.: A study of the effect of limitation of food intake and the method of feeding on the rate of weight gain during hypothalamic obesity in the albino rat. Amer. J. Physiol., 147:695-707, 1946.

Bruch, H.: Hunger and instinct. J. Nerv. Ment. Dis., 149:91-114, 1969.

Carlisle, H. J., and Stellar, E.: Caloric regulation and food preference in normal, hyperphagic, and aphagic rats. J. Comp. Physiol. Psychol., 69:107-114, 1969.

Cohn, C., and Joseph, D.: Influence of body weight and body fat on appetite of "normal" lean and obese rats. Yale J. Biol. Med., 34:598-607, 1962.

Corbett, S. W.: Energy balance in the lateral hypothalamically lesioned rat. M. S. Thesis, University of Wisconsin, Madison, 1979.

Cruce, J. A. F., Greenwood, M. R. C., Johnson, P. R., et al.: Genetic versus hypothalamic obesity: Studies of intake and dietary manipulations in rats. J. Comp. Physiol. Psychol., 87:295-301, 1974.

Cunningham, D. J., and Cabanac, M.: Evidence from behavioral thermo-regulatory responses of a shift in set-point temperature related to the menstrual cycle. J. Physiol., 63:236-238, 1971.

deCastro, J., Paullin, S. & DeLugas, G.: Insulin and Glucagon As determinants of body weight set point and microregulation in rats. J. Comp. Physiol. Psychol. 92, 571-579, 1978.

Durnin, J. V. G. A.: Appetite and the relationships between expenditure and intake of calories in man. J. Physiol. (Lond.), 156:294-306, 1961.

Edholm, O. G., Fletcher, J. G., Widdowson, E. M., et al.: The energy expenditure and food intake of individual men. Brit. J. Nutr., 9:286-300, 1955.

Ellison, G. D.: Behaviour and the balance between norepinephrine and serotonin. Acta. Neurobiol. Exp., 35:499-515, 1975.

Ellison, G. D., and Sorenson, C. A.: Two feeding syndromes following surgical isolation of the hypothalamus in rats. J. Comp. Physiol. Psychol., 70:173-188, 1970.

Engelberg, J.: Physiological regulation: The steady state. The Physiologist, 9:69-88, 1966.

Epstein, L. H., Wing, R. R., and Thompson, J. K.: The relationship between exercise intensity, caloric intake and weight. Addict. Behav. 3:185-190, 1978.

Faust, I. M., Johnson, P. R., and Hirsch, J.: Dietary induction of adipocyte number increase in the adult rat. Second International Congress on Obesity, Washington, 1977.

Faust, I., Johnson, P., Stern, J., et al.: Diet-induced adipocyte number increase in adult rats: a new model of obesity. Amer. J. Physiol., 235(3):E279-E286, 1978.

Forbes, E. G., Kriss, M., and Miller, R. C.: The energy metabolism of the albino rat in relation to the plane of nutrition. J. Nutr., 8:535-552, 1934.

Gale, S. K., and Sclafani, A.: Comparison of ovarian and hypothalamic obesity syndromes in the female rat: Effects of diet palatability on food intake and body weight. J. Comp. Physiol. Psychol., 91:381-392, 1977.

Gale, S. K., Van Itallie, T. B., and Faust, I. M.: Effects of palatable diets on body weight and adipose tissue cellularity in the adult obese female Zucker rat (fa/fa). Metabolism, in press, 1980.

Goodner, C. J., and Ogilvie, J. T.: Homeostasis of body weight in a diabetes clinic population. Diabetes, 23:318-326, 1974.

Grafe, E., and Graham, D.: Uber die Anpassungsfahigkeit des tierschen Organismus an uberreichliche Nahringszufuhr. Ztschr, f. Physiol. Chem., Strassb., 73:1-67, 1911.

Greenwood, M. R. C., Quartermain, D., Johnson, P. R., et al.: Food motivated behavior in genetically obese and hypothalamic-hyperphagic rats and mice. Physiol. Behav., 13:687-692, 1974.

Grossman, S. P.: A neuropharmacological analysis of hypothalamic and extrahypothalamic mechanisms concerned with the regulation of food and water intake. Ann. New York Acad. Sci. 157:902-912, 1969.

Grossman, S. P.: Role of the hypothalamus in the regulation of food and water intake. Psychol. Rev., 82:200-224, 1975.

Hammel, H. T.: Neurons and temperature regulation. In Yamamoto, W. S., and Brobeck, J. R., eds.: Physiological Controls and Regulations. Philadelphia, W. B. Saunders Co., 1965.

Heffner, T. G., Zigmond, M. J., and Stricker, E. M.: Effects of dopaminergic agonists and antagonists on feeding in intact and 6-hydroxy-dopamine-treated rats. J. Pharm. Exper. Ther., 201:386-399, 1977.

Hetherington, A. W.: The production of hypothalamic obesity in rats already displaying chronic hypopituitarism. Amer. J. Physiol., 140:89-92, 1943.

Hoebel, B. G., and Teitelbaum, P.: Weight regulation in normal and hypo-thalamic hyperphagic rats. J. Comp. Physiol. Psychol., 61:189-193, 1966.

David R. Jacobs, Jr., and Sara Gottenborg, "Smoking and Weight," American Journal of Public Health 71 (1981):391-96; idem, "Smokers Eat More, Weigh Less than Nonsmokers." American Journal of Public Health 71, 859-60, 1981.

Richard E. Keesey, "A Set-Point Analysis of the Regulation of Body Weight," in Stunkard, Obesity, pp. 144-65.

Kanarek, R. B., and Hirsch, E.: Dietary-induced overeating in experimental animals. Fed. Proc., 36:154-158, 1977.

Kratz, C. M., and Levitsky, D. A.: Dietary obesity: differential effects with self-selection and composite diet feeding techniques. Physiol. Behav., 22:245-249, 1979.

Lemonnier, D.: Effect of age, sex, and site on the cellularity of the adipose tissue in mice and rats rendered obese by a high fat diet. J. Clin. Nutr., 51:2907-2915, 1972.

Keesey, R. E., Boyle, P. D., Kemnitz, J. W., et al.: The role of the lateral hypothalamus in determining the body weight set-point. In Novin, D., Wyrwicka, W., and Bray, G. A., eds.: Hunger: Basic Mechanisms and Clinical Implications. Raven Press, New York, 1976.

Keesey, R. E., Boyle, P. C., and Storlien, L. H.: Food intake and utilization in lateral hypothalamically lesioned rats. Physiol. Behav., 21:265-268, 1978.

Kennedy, G. C.: The role of depot fat in the hypothalamic control of food intake in the rat. Proc. Roy. Soc., Series B, 140:578-592, 1953.

Leibowitz, S. F.: Ingestion in the satiated rat: role of alpha and beta receptors in mediating effects of hypothalamic adrenergic stimulation. Physiol. Behav., 14:743-754, 1975.

Leibowitz, S. F., and Papadakos, P. J.: Serotonin-Norepinephrine interaction in the paraventricular nucleus: antagonistic effects on feeding behavior in the rat. Neurosci. Abstr., 4:177, 1978.

Le Magnen, J., Devos, M., Gaudilliere, J. P., et al.: Role of a lipostatic mechanism in regulation by feeding of energy balance in rats. J. Comp. Physiol. Psychol. 84:1-23, 1973.

Levitsky, D. A., Faust, I., and Glassman, M.: The ingestion of food and the recovery of body weight following fasting in the naive rat. Physiol. Behav., 17:575-580, 1965.

Liebelt, R. A., Ichinoe, S., and Nicholson, N.: Regulatory influences of adipose tissue on food intake and body weight. Ann. N.Y. Acad. Sci., 131:559-582, 1965.

Maxfield, E., and Konishi, F.: Patterns of food intake and physical activity in obesity. J. Amer. Dietet. Assoc., 49:406-408, 1966.

Mayer, J.: Regulation of energy intake and the body weight. The glucostatic theory and the lipostatic hypothesis. Ann. N.Y. Acad. Sci., 63:15-43, 1955.

Mayer, J., Roy, P., and Mitra, K. P.: Relation between caloric intake, body weight, and physical work: Studies in an industrial male population in West Bengal. Amer. J. Clin. Nutr., 4:169-175, 1956.

Miller, D. S., and Mumford, P.: Luxuskonsumption. In Apfelbaum, M., ed.: Energy Balance in Man. Paris, Masson et Cie, 1973.

Mitchel, J. S., and Keesey, R. E.: Defense of a lowered weight maintenance level by lateral hypothalamically lesioned rats: Evidence from a restriction-refeeding regimen. Physiol. Behav., 18:1121-1125, 1977.

Mogenson, G. J.: Changing views of the role of the hypothalamus in the control of ingestive behaviors. In Lederis, K., and Cooper, K. E., eds.: Recent Studies of Hypothalamic Function. Basel, S. Karger, 1974.

Mrosovsky, N., and Powley, T. L.: Set-points for body weight and fat. Behav. Biol., 20:205-223, 1977.

Muto, S., and Miyhara, C.: Eating behavior of young rats: experiments on selective feeding of diet and sugar solutions. Brit. J. Nutr., 28:327-337, 1972.

Newsholme, E.A.: A possible metabolic basis for the control of body weight. New Engl. J. Med. 302, 400-405, 1980.

Nisbett, R. E.: Hunger, obesity, and the ventromedial hypothalamus. Psychol. Rev., 79:433-453, 1972.

Nisbett, R.E.: Taste, deprivation, and weight determinants of eating behavior. J. Personality Soc. Psychol. 10, 107-116, 1978.

Novin, D., Sanderson, J. D. & Gonzales, M.: Feeding after nutrient infusions: effects of hypothalamic lesions and vagotomy. Physiol. Behav. 22, 107-113, 1979.

Novin, D., and Vander Weele, D. A.: Visceral involvement in feeding: there is more to regulation than the hypothalamus. In Sprague, J. M. and Epstein, A. N., eds.: Progress in Psychobiology and Physiological Psychology. Vol. 7. New York, Academic Press, 1977.

Parameswaran, S. V., Steffens, A. B., Hervey, G. R., et al.: Involvement of a humoral factor in regulation of body weight in parabiotic rats. Amer. J. Physiol., 232:R150-R157, 1977.

Peck, Jeffrey W., Rats Defend Different Body Weights Depending on Palatability and Accessibility of Their Food, Journal of Comparative and Physiological Psychology 92: 555-70, 1978.

Pitts, G. C., and Bull, L. S.: Exercise, dietary obesity, and growth in the rat. Amer. J. Physiol., 232-R38-R44, 1977.

Planansky, K.: Changes in weight in patients receiving a tranquillizing drug. Psychiatr. Quart., 32:289-292, 1958.

Polivy, J., Herman, C. P., and Warsh, S.: Internal and external components of emotionality in restrained and unrestrained eaters, J. Abnorm. Psychol., 87:497-504, 1978.

Porikos, K., Booth, G. R., and Van Itallie, T. B.: Effect of covert nutritive dilution on the spontaneous food intake of obese individuals: a pilot study. Amer. J. Clin. Nutr., 30:1638-1644, 1977.

Powley, T. L.: The ventromedial hypothalamic syndrome, satiety, and a cephalic phase hypothesis. Psychol. Rev., 84:89-126, 1977.

Powley, T. L., and Keesey, R. E.: Relationship of body weight to the lateral hypothalamic feeding syndrome. J. Comp. Physiol. Psychol., 70:25-36, 1970.

Powley, T. L., Opsahl, C. A., Cox, J. E., et al.: The role of the hypothalamus in energy homeostasis. In Morgane, P. J., and Panksepp, J., eds.: Handbook of the Hypothalamus. New York, Marcel Dekker & Co., 1978.

Rabin, B. M: Ventromedial hypothalamic control of food intake and satiety: A reappraisal. Brain Res., 43:317-324, 1972.

Rodin, J.: Obesity: why the losing battle? Master Lecture Series. Washington DC: American Psychological Association, 1977.

Rodin, J.: The effects of obesity and set point on taste responsiveness and intake in humans. J. Comp. Physiol. Psychol., 89:1003-1009, 1975.

Rodin, J.: The role of perception of internal and external signals on regulation of feeding in overweight and nonobese individuals. In Silverstone, T., ed.: Appetite and Food Intake. Braunschweig. Pergamon Press/Vieweg, 1976.

Rolls, B. J. & Rowe, E. A.: Dietary obesity: permanent changes in body weight. J. Physiol. 272, 2P, 1977.

Rolls, E. T., and Rolls, B. J.: Activity of neurones in sensory, hypothalamic and motor areas during feeding in the monkey. In Katsuki, Y., Sato, M., Takagi, S. F., et al., eds.: Food Intake and Chemical Senses, Tokyo, University of Tokyo Press, 1977.

Romsos, D. R., Hornshuh, M. J., and Leveille, G. A.: Influence of dietary fat and carbohydrate on food intake, body weight and body fat of adult dogs. Proc. Soc. Exper. Biol. Med., 157:278-281, 1978.

Ross, M. H.: Protein, calories and life expectance. Fed. Proc., 18:1190-1206, 1959.

Rothwell, N. J., and Stock, M. J.: Mechanisms of weight gain and loss in reversible obesity in the rat. J. Physiol., 276:6OP-61P, 1978.

Ruderman, A. J. & Wilson, G. T.: Weight restraint, cognitions and counterregulation. Behav. Res. Ther. 16, 581-590, 1979.

Sclafani, A., and Springer, D.: Dietary obesity in adult rats: Similarities to hypothalamic and human obesity syndromes. Physiol. Behav., 17:461-471, 1976.

Silverstone, T., ed.: Appetite and Food Intake. Report of the Dahlen Workshop on Appetite and Food Intake. Life Sciences Research Reports, Berlin, 1971.

Sims, E. A. H., and Horton, E. S.: Endocrine and metabolic adaptation to obesity and starvation. Amer. J. Clin. Nutr., 21:1455-1470, 1968.

Spiegel, T. A.: Caloric regulation of food intake in man. J. Comp. Physiol. Psychol., 81:24-37, 1973.

Smith, G. P., and Gibbs, J.: Postprandial satiety. In Sprague, J. M. and Epstein, A. N., eds.: Progress in Psychobiology and Physiological Psychology. Vol. 8. New York, Academic Press, 1979.

Stephanie, P. A., Heald, F. P., and Mayer, J.: Caloric intake in relation to energy output of obese and nonobese adolescent boys. Amer. J. Clin. Nutr., 7:55-62, 1959.

Stern, J. S., Dunn, J. R., and Johnson, P. R.: Effects of exercise on the development of obesity in obese yellow mice. Presented at the Second International Congress on Obesity, Washington, D.C., October, 1977.

Stricker, E. M., and Zigmond, M. J.: Brain catecholamines and the lateral hypothalamic syndrome. In Novin, D., Wyrwicka, W., and Bray, G., eds.: Hunger: Basic Mechanisms and Clinical Implications. New York, Raven Press, 1976.

Stunkard, A. J.: Environment and obesity: recent advances in our understanding of the regulation of food intake in man. Fed. Proc., 27:1367-1373, 1968.

Szepesi, B.: A model of nutritionally induced overweight: Weight "rebound" following caloric restriction. In Bray, G. A., ed.: Recent Advances in Obesity Research. Vol. 2. London, Newman, Ltd., 1978.

Teitelbaum, P.: Disturbances in feeding and drinking behavior after hypothalamic lesions. In Jones, M. A., ed.: Nebraska Symposium on Motivation, 1961, Lincoln, University Nebraska Press, 1961.

Teitelbaum, P., and Epstein, A. N.: The lateral hypothalamic syndrome: Recovery of feeding and drinking after lateral hypothalamic lesions. Psychol. Rev., 69:74-94, 1962.

Teitelbaum, P., and Wolgin, D. L.: Neurotransmitters and the regulation of food intake. In Gispen, W. H., Van Wimersma Greidanus, T. B., Bohus, B., and de Wied, D., eds.: Progress in Brain Research: Hormones, Homeostasis and the Brain. Amsterdam, Elsevier Scientific Publ., Vol. 42, 1975.

Trygstad, O., Foss. I., Edminson, P., et al.: Humoral control of appetite: a urinary anorexigenic peptide. Chromatographic patters of urinary peptides in anorexia nervosa. Acta Endocrinol., 89:196-208, 1978.

Vague, J., and Boyer, J., eds.: The regulation of the adipose tissue mass. Proceedings of the IVth International Meeting of Endocrinology. Amsterdam, Excerpta Medica, 1974.

VanderWeele, D. A., Geiselman, P. J. & Novin, D.: Pancreatic glucagon, food deprivation and feeding in intact and vagotomized rabbits. Physiol. Behav. 23, 155-158, 1979.

Van der Gugten, J., de Kloet, E. R., Versteeg, D. H. G., and Slangen, J. L.: Regional hypothalamic catecholamine metabolism and feeding. Sixth International Conference on the Physiology of Food and Fluid Intake Abstracts. Paris-Jouy en Josas (France), 1977.

Waxman, M., and Stunkard, A. J.: Caloric intake and expenditure of obese children. J. Pediat., 96:187-193, 1980.

Wilkinson, P., Parklin, J., Pearloom, G. et al.: Enerqy intake and physical activity in obese children. Brit. Med. J., 1:756, 1977.

Wirtshafter, D., and Davis, J. D.: Set-points, settling points, and the control of body weight. Physiol. Behav., 19:75-78, 1977.

Wolgin, D. L., Cytawa, J., and Teitelbaum, P.: The role of activation in the regulation of food intake. In Novin, D., Whrwicka, W., and Bray, G., eds.: Hunger: Basic Mechanisms and Clinical Implications. New York, Raven Press, 1976.

Woods, S. C., McKay, L. D., Stein, L. J., West, D. B., Lotter, E. C. & Porte, D.: Neuroendocrine regulation of food intake and body weight. Brain Res. Bull. 5, Suppl. 4, 1-5, 1980.

Woods, S. C., and Porte, D., Jr.: Insulin and the set-point regulation of body weight. In Novin, D., Whrwicka, W., and Bray, G., eds.: Hunger: Basic Mechanisms and Clinical Implications, New York, Raven Press, 1976.

Wooley, S. C.: Physiologic versus cognitive factors in short term food regulation in the obese and nonobese. Psychosom. Med., 34:62-68, 1972.

Zigmond, M. J., and Stricker, E. M.: Recovery of feeding and drinking by rats after intraventricular 6-hydroxydopamine or lateral hypothalamic lesions. Science, 182:717-719, 1973.

Regulation of Eating, Appetite, and Satiety

Anika, S. M., Haupt, T. R. & Haupt, K. A.: Satiety elicited by cholecystokinin in intact and vagotomized rats. Physiol. Behav. 19, 761-766, 1977.

Antin, J., Gibbs, J., Holt, J., et al.: Cholecystokinin elicits the complete behavioural sequence of satiety in rats. J. Comp. Physiol. Psychol., 89:784-790, 1975.

Ashley, D. V. M., Coscina, D. V., and Anderson, G. H.: Selective decrease in protein intake following brain serotonin depletion. Life Sci., 24:973-984, 1979.

Booth, D. A.: Conditioned satiety in the rat. J. Comp. Physiol. Psychol. 81, 457-471, 1972.

Booth, D. A., Toates, F. M., and Platt, S. V.: Control system for hunger and its implications in animals and man. In Novin D., Wyrwicka, W., and Bray, G. A., eds.: Hunger: Basic Mechanisms and Clinical Implications. New York, Raven Press, 1976.

Booth, D. A.: Caloric compensation in rats with continuous or intermittent access to food. Physiol. Behav., 8:891-899, 1972.

Booth, D. A.: Approaches to feeding control. In Silverstone, T., ed.: Appetite and Food Intake. Berlin, Abakon, 1976.

Booth, D. A.: Appetite and satietyas metabolic expectancies. In Katsuki, Y., Sato, M., Takagi, S. F., et al.: Food Intake and Chemical Senses. Tokyo, University of Tokyo Press, 1977.

Booth, D. A.: First steps toward an integrated quantitative approach to human feeding and obesity with some implications for research into treatment. In Bray, G. A., ed.: Recent Advances in Obesity Research II. London, Newman, 1978.

Booth, D. A.: Prediction of feeding behaviour from energy flows in the rat. In Booth, D. A., ed.: Hunger Models: Computable Theroy of Feeding Control. London, Academic Press, 1978.

Booth, D. A.: Metabolism and the control of feeding in man and animals. In Brown, K., and Cooper, S. J., eds.: Chemical Influences on Behaviour. London, Academic Press, 1978.

Booth, D. A., and Campbell, C. S.: Relation of fatty acids to feeding behaviour. Physiol. Behav., 15:523-535, 1975.

Booth, D. A., Chase, A., and Campbell, A. T.: Relative effectiveness of protein in the late stages of appetite suppression in man. Physiol. Behav., 5:1299-1302, 1970.

Booth, D. A., and Davis, J. D.: Gastrointestinal factors in the acquisition of oral sensory control of satiation. Physiol. Behav., 11:23-29, 1973.

Booth, D. A., and Jarman, S. P.: Inhibition of food intake in the rat following complete absorption of glucose delivered into the stomach, intestine or liver. J. Physiol. (Lond)., 259:501-522, 1976.

Booth, D. A.: Satiety and behavioral caloric compensation following intragastric glucose loads in the rat. J. Comp. Physiol. Psychol., 78: 412-432, 1972.

Bray, G. A.: Peripheral metabolic factors in the regulation of feeding. In Appetite and food intake, ed T. Silverstone, pp. 141-176. Berlin: Abakon Verlagsgesellschaft, 1976.

Brobeck, J. R.: Nature of satiety signals. Am. J. Clin. Nutr. 28, 806-807, 1975.

Cohn, C. & Joseph, D.: Changes in body composition with force feeding. Am. J. Physiol. 196, 965-968, 1959.

Cook, A. I. & Shields, R.: The effect of trunical vagotomy and drainage on the duodenal osmoreceptor control of gastric emptying. Br. J. Surg, Res. 63, 657-658, 1976.

Davis, J. D., Collins, B. J., and Levine, M. W.: The interaction between gustatory stimulation and gut feedback in the control of the ingestion of liquid diets. In Booth, D. A., ed.: Hunger Models: Computable Theory of Feeding Control. London, Academic Press, 1978.

Davis, J. D. & Campbell, C. S.: Peripheral control of meal size in the rat: effect of sham feeding on meal size and drinking rate. J. Comp Physiol. Psychol. 83, 379-387, 1973.

Davis, J. D. & Campbell, C. S.: Distention of the small intestines, satiety and the control of food intake. Am. J. Clin. Nutr. 31, S255-S258, 1978.

Debons, A. F., Krimsky, I., From, A. & Cloutier, R. J.: Rapid effects of insulin on the hypothalamic satiety center. Am. J. Physiol. 217, 1114-1118, 1969.

Deutsch, J. A., Young, W. G. & Kalogeris, T. J.: The stomach signals satiety. Science 201, 165-167.

Deutsch, J. A.: The stomach in food satiation and the regulation of appetite. Prog. Neurobiol. 10, 135-153, 1978.

Deutsch, J. A., Gonzalez, M. F. & Young, W. G.: Two factors control meal size. Brain Res. Bull. 5, Suppl. 4, 55-57, 1980.

Ehman, G. K., Albert, D. J. & Jamieson, J. J.: Injections into the duodenum and the induction of satiety in the rat. Can. J. Psychol. 25, 147-166, 1971.

Gibbs, J., Young, R. D. & Smith, G. P.: Cholecystokinin decreases food intake in rats. J. Comp. Physiol. Psychol. 84, 488-495, 1973.

Goldman, J. K., Bernardis, L. L. & Frohman, L. A.: Food intake in hypothalamic obesity. Am. J. Physiol. 227, 88-91, 1976.

Grossman, S. P.: Role of hypothalamus in the regulation of food and water intake. Psychol. Rev. 82, 200-224, 1975.

Hamilton, C. L.: Rat's preference for high fat diets. J. Comp. Physiol. Psychol., 58:459-460, 1964.

Harris, L. J., Clay, J., Hargreaves, F. J., et al.: Appetite and choice of diet. The ability of the vitamin B deficient rat to discriminate between diets containing and lacking the vitamin. Proc. Roy. Soc. B., 113:161-190, 1933.

Holman, G. L.: Intragastric reinforcement effect. J. Comp. Physiol. Psychol., 69:432-441, 1969.

Hunt, J. N. A.: A possible relation between the regulation of gastric emptying and food intake. Am. J. Physiol. 239, G1-G4, 1980.

Janowitz, H. D.: Role of the gastrointestinal tract in the regulation of food intake. In Code, C. F., ed.: Handbook of Physiology: Alimentary Canal, I. Washington, D.C., American Physiological Society, 1967,

Johansson, C. & Ekelund, K.: Relation between body weight and the gastric and intestinal handling of an oral calorie load. Gut 17, 456-462, 1976.

Kanarek, R. B., and Hirsch, E.: Dietary-induced overeating in experimental animals. Fed. Proc., 36:154-158, 1977.

Keys, A., Brozek, J., Henschel, A., et al.: The Biology of Human Starvation. Minneapolis, University of Minnesota Press, 1950.

Koopmans, H. S.: Jejunal signals in hunger satiety. Behav. Biol. 14, 309-324, 1975.

Koopmans, H. S.: Regulation of food intake during long-term loss of food from the intestines. Proc. Soc. Exper. Biol. Med. 157, 430-434, 1978.

Koopmans, H. S., Sclafani, A., Fichtner, C. & Aravich, P.: The effects of ileal transposition on food intake and body weight loss in VMH-obese rats. Am. J. Clin. Nutr. (In press), 1981.

Kraly, F. S. & Smith, G. P.: Combined pregastric and gastric stimulation by food is sufficient for normal meal size. Physiol. Behav. 21, 405-408, 1978.

Liebling, D. S., Eisner, J. D., Gibbs, J. & Smith, G. P.: Intestinal satiety in rats. J. Comp. Physiol. Psychol. 89, 955-965, 1975.

Lepkovsky, S., Simick, M. K., Furuta, F., Feldman, S. E. & Park, R.: Stomach and upper intestine of the rat in the regulation of food intake. J. Nutr. 12, 1491-1499, 1975.

LeMagnen, J.: Sweet preference and the sensory control of caloric intake. In Weiffenbach, J. M., ed.: Taste and Development: The Genesis of Sweet Preference. Washington, DC, US Gov't. Printing Office, 1977.

LeMagnen, J.: Hunger and food palatability in the control of feeding behaviour. In Katsuki, Y., Sato, M., Takagi, S. F., et al.: Food intake and chemical senses. Tokyo, University of Tokyo Press, 1977.

Levitsky, D. A. & Collier, G.: Effects of diet and deprivation on meal eating behavior in rats. Physiol. Behav. 3, 137-140, 1968.

Lorenz, D., Gibbs, J. & Smith, G. P.: Effect of cholecystokinin and other gut hormones on sham feeding in the rat. In Gut hormones, ed. S. R. Bloom, pp. 224-226. London: Churchill Livingstone, 1978.

Marshall, J. F.: Neurochemistry of central monoamine systems as related to food intake. In Silverstone, T., ed.: Appetite and Food Intake. Dahlem Konferenzen, Berlin, 1976.

McHugh. P. R. & Moran, T. H.: Calories and gastric emptying: a regulatory capacity with implications for feeding. Am. J. Physiol. 236, R254-R260, 1979.

McHugh, P. R., Moran, T. H. & Barton, G. N.: Satiety: a graded behavioral phenomenon regulating caloric intake. Science 190, 167-169, 1975.

Metzner, H. L., Lamphear, D. E. Wheeler, N. C., et al.: The relationship between frequency of eating and adiposity in adult men and women in the Tecumseh Community Health Study. Amer. J. Clin. Nutr. 30:712-715, 1977.

Meyer, J. E.: Psychopathology and eating disorders. In Silverstone, T., ed.: Appetite and Food Intake. Berlin, Abakon, 1976.

Myers, R. D. & McCaleb, M. L.: Feeding: satiety signal from intestine triggers brain's noradrenergic mechanism. Science 209, 1035-1037, 1980.

Miller, D. S. & Mumford, P.: Gluttony 1. An experimental study of overeating on high or low protein diets. Am. J. Clin. Nutr. 20, 1212-1222, 1967.

Miller, D. S. & Payne, P. R.: Weight maintenance and food intake. J. Nutr. 78, 255-262, 1962.

Mogenson, G. J., and Avrith, D.: The use of colchicine as a reversible blocker to investigate the control of food intake and body weight regulations. In Katsuki, Y., Sato, M., Takagi, S. F., et al.: Food Intake and Chemical Senses. Tokyo, University of Tokyo Press, 1977.

Novin, D.: Visceral mechanisms in the control of food intake. In Hunger: basic mechanisms and clinical implications, ed D. Novin, W. Wyrwicka & G. Bray, pp. 357-367. New York, Raven Press, 1976.

Novin, D., Wyrwicka, W., and Bray, G.: Hunger: Basic Mechanisms and Clinical Implications. New York, Raven Press, 1976.

Novin, D., VanderWeele, D. A. & Rezek, M.: Infusion of 2-deoxy-d-glucose into the hepatic-portal system causes eating: evidence for peripheral glucoreceptors. Science 181,858-860, 1973.

Oomura, Y.: Significance of glucose insulin and free fatty acid on the hypothalamic feeding and satiety neurons. In Novin, D., Wyrwicka, W., and Bray, G., eds.: Hunger: Basic Mechanisms and Clinical Implications. New York, Raven Press, 1976.

Oscai, L. B., and McGarr, J. A.: Evidence that the amount of food consumed in early life fixes appetite in the rat. Amer. J. Physiol., 235:R141-R144, 1978.

Oscai, L. B.: Evidence that size does not determine voluntary food intake in the rat. Am. J. Physiol. 238. E318-E321, 1980.

Panksepp, J., and Nance, D. M.: Insulin, glucose and hypothalamic regulation of feeding. Physiol. Behav. 9:447-451, 1972.

Polivy, J.: Perception of calories and regulation of intake in restrained and unrestrained subjects. Addict. Behav., 1:237-243, 1976.

Rezek, M. & Kroeger, E. A.: Glucose antimetabolites and hunger (theoretical article). J. Nutr. 106, 145-157, 1976.

Rodin, J.: The relationship between external responsiveness and the development and maintenance of obesity. In Novin, D., Wyrwicka, W., and Bray, G., eds.: Hunger: Basic Mechanisms and Clinical Implications. New York, Raven Press, 1976.

Rolls, B. J., Rolls, E. T. & Row, E. A.: Sensory specific satiety and appetite. Int. J. Obesity 3, 397-398, 1979.

Russek, M.: Demonstration of the influence on an hepatic glucose sensitive mechanism on food intake. Physiol. Behav. 5, 1207-1209, 1970.

Sclafani, A.: Appetite and hunger in experimental obesity syndromes. In Novin, D., Wyrwicka, W., and Bray, G., eds: Hunger: Basic Mechanisms and Clinical Implications. New York, Raven Press, 1976, pp. 281-295.

Sclafani, A.: Neural pathways involved in the ventromedial hypothalamic lesion syndrome in the rat. J. Comp. Physiol. Psychol., 77:70-96, 1971.

Silverstone, T.: Appetite and Food Intake. Berlin, Dahlem Konferenzen, 1976.

Smith, G. P. & Cushin, B. J.: Cholecystokinin acts in a vagally innervated abdominal site to elicit satiety. Soc. Neurosci. 4, 180, 1978.

Smith, G. P. & Gibbs, J.: Postprandial Satiety. In Progress in physiological psychology and psychobiology. ed J. D. Sprague & A. N. Epstein, pp. 179-242. New York, Academic Press, 1979.

Smith, G. P. & Gibbs, J.: What the gut tells the brain about feeding behavior. In Appetite and food intake, ed T. Silverstone, pp. 129-139. Berlin, Abakon Verlagsgesellschaft, 1976.

Smith, M., Pool, R. & Weinberg, H.: The role of bulk in the control of eating. J. Comp. Physiol. Psychol. 55, 115-120, 1962.

Smith, P. G., and Epstein, A. N.: Increased feeding response to decreased glucose utilization in the rat and monkey. Amer. J. Physiol., 217:1083-1087, 1969.

Snowden, C. T.: Production of satiety with small intraduodenal infusions in the rat. J. Comp. Physiol. 88, 231-238, 1975.

Snowdon, C. T.: Gastrointestinal sensory and motor control of food intake. J. Comp. Physiol. Psychol., 71:68-76, 1970.

Steffens, A. B.: Influence of reversible obesity on eating behavior, blood glucose, and insulin in the rat. Am. J. Physiol. 228, 1738-1744, 1975.

Strubbe, J. H., Steffens, A. B. & deRuiter, L.: Plasma insulin and the time pattern of feeding in the rat. Physiol. Behav. 18, 81-86, 1977.

Tepperman, J. & Tepperman, H. M.: Adaptive hyperlipogenesis - late 1964 model. Ann. N.Y. Acad. Sci. 131, 404-411, 1965.

VanderWeele, D. A. & Sanderson, J. D.: Peripheral glucosensitive satiety in the rabbit and the rat. In Hunger: basic mechanisms and clinical implications, eds D. Novin, W. Wyrwicka & G. Bray. pp. 383-393. New York, Raven Press, 1976.

VanderWeele, D. A., Haraczkiewicz, E. & Van Itallie, T. B.: Elevated insulin level as a putative satiety signal in obese and normal-weight rats. Appetite (In press), 1981.

VanderWeele, D. A., Novin, D., Rezek, M. & Sanderson, J. D.: Duodenal or hepatic-portal glucose perfusion: Evidence for duodenally based satiety. Physiol. Behav. 12, 467-473, 1974;

VanderWeele, D. A., Pi-Sunyer, F. X., Novin, D. & Bush, M. J.: Chronic insulin infusion suppresses food ingestion and body weight gain in rats. Brain Res. Bull. 5, Suppl. 4, 7-11, 1980.

Van Itallie, T. B., Gale, S. K., and Kissileff, H. R.: Control of food intake in the regulation of depot fat: An overview. In Katzen, H. M., and Mahler, R. J., eds.: Diabetes, Obesity and Vascular Disease. Vol 2. Halstead, New York, 1978.

Wade, G. N., and Zucker, I.: Development of hormonal control over food intake and body weight in female rats. J. Comp. Physiol. Psychol., 70:213-220, 1970.

Wilmshurst, P. & Crawley, J. C. W.: The measurement of gastric transit time in obese subjects using 24Na and the effects of energy content and guar gum on gastric emptying and satiety. Br. J. Nutr. 44, 1-6, 1980.

Woo, R., Kissileff, H. R. & Pi-Sunyer, F. X.: Is insulin a satiety hormone? Fed. Proc. 38, 547, 1979.

Regulation of Energy Balance

Andrews, F. & Jackson, F.: Increasing fatness inversely related to increase in metabolic rate but directly related to decrease in deep body temperature in young men and women during cold exposure. Ir. J. Med. Sci. 147, 329-330, 1978.

Apfelbaum, M.: Influence of level of energy intake on energy expenditure in man. In Bray, G. A., ed.: Obesity in Perspective. Washington, D.C., U.S. Government Printing Office, 1972.

Apfelbaum, M., Bostsarron, J., and Lacatis, D.: Effect of calorie restriction and excessive caloric intake on energy expenditure. Amer. J. Clin. Nutr., 24:1405-1409, 1971.

Ball, E. G. & Jungas, R. L.: On the action of hormones which accelerate the rate of oxygen consumption and fatty acid release in rat adipose tissue in vitro. Proc. Natn. Acad. Sci. U.S.A. 47,932-941, 1961.

Blaza, S. E.: Thermogenesis in lean and obese individuals. PhD Thesis, CNAA. Also: Blaza, S. E. & Garrow, J. S. In preparation, 1980.

Blaza, S. E. & Garrow, J. S.: The thermogenic response to comfortable temperature extremes in lean and obese subjects. Proc. Nut. Soc. 39, 85A, 1981.

Bray, G. A.: Effect of caloric restriction on energy expenditure in obese patients. Lancet, 2:397-398, 1969.

Bray, G. A.: Oxygen consumption of genetically obese rats. Experientia, 25:1100-1101, 1969.

Bray, G. A.: Metabolic and regulatory obesity in rats and man. Hormones Metabol. Res., 2:175-180, 1970.

Boyle, P. C., Storlien, L. H., and Keesey, R. E.: Increased efficiency of food utilization following weight loss. Physiol. Behav., 21:261-264, 1978.

Bullen, B., Reed, R. & Mayer, R.: Physical activity of obese and non obese adolescent girls appraised by motion picture sampling. J. Clin. Nutr. 14-211, 1964.

Brooks, S. L., Rothwell, N. J. & Stock, M. J.: The effects of hypoxia on diet-induced thermogenesis in the rat. J. Physiol. 203, 35P, 1980.

Brooks, S. L., Rothwell, N. J., Stock, M. J., Goodbody, A. E. & Trayhurn, P.: Increased proton conductance pathway in brown adipose tissue mitochondria of rats exhibiting diet-induced thermogenesis. Nature 286, 274-276, 1980.

Burskirk, E. R., Thompson, R. H., Lutwak, L., et al.: Energy balance of obese patients during weight reduction: Influence of diet restriction and exercise. Ann. New York Acad. Sci., 110:918-940, 1963.

Burskirk, E. R., Thompson, R. H., & Whedon, G. D.: Metabolic response to cold air in men and women in relation to total body fat content. J. Appl. Physiol. 18, 603-612, 1963.

Danforth, E., Burger, A. G., Goldman, R. F. & Sims, E. A. H.: Thermogenesis during weight gain. In Recent advances in obesity research: II, ed G. A. Gray, pp. 229-238. Newman, London, 1978.

Dauncey, M. J.: Energy metabolism in man and the influence of diet and temperature: a review. J. Hum. Nutr. 33, 259-269, 1979.

Dore, C., Hesp, R., Wilkins, D. & Garrow, J. S.: A standard for resting metabolic rate in obese women. (In preparation), 1980.

Foster, D. O. & Frydman, M. L.: Nonshivering thermogenesis in the rat. Measurements of blood flow with microspheres point to brown adipose tissue as the dominant site of calorigenesis induced by noradrenaline. Can. J. Physiol. Pharmac. 56, 110-122, 1978.

Foster, D. O. & Frydman, M. L.: Tissue distribution of cold-induced thermogenesis in conscious warm- or cold-acclimated rats re-evaluated from changes in tissue blood flow: the dominant role of brown adipose tissue in the replacement of shivering by non-shivering thermogenesis. Can. J. Physiol. Pharmac. 57, 257-270, 1979.

Foster, D. O. & Frydman, M. L.: Non-shivering thermogenesis in the rat. II. Measurements of blood flow with microspheres point to brown adipose tissue as the dominant site of the calorigenesis induced by noradrenaline. Can. J. Physiol. Pharmac, 56, 110-122, 1978.

Garrow, J. S.: Energy Balance and Obesity in Man. Amsterdam, North Holland, 1978.

Garrow, J. S.: The regulation of energy expenditure in man. In Bray, G. A., ed.: Recent Advances in Obesity Research II. Newman, London, 1978.

Garrow, J. S. & Hawes, S. F.: The role of amino acid oxidation in causing specific dynamic action in man. Br. J. Nutr. 27, 211-219, 1972.

Glick, Z., Shvartz, E., Magazanik, A. & Modan, M.: Absence of increased thermogenesis during short-term overfeeding in normal and overweight women. Am. J. Clin. Nutr. 30, 1026-1035, 1977.

Heaton, I. M.: The distribution of brown adipose tissue in the human. J. Anat. 112, 35-39, 1972.

Himms-Hagen, J. & Desautels, M.: A mitochondrial defect in brown adipose tissue of the obese (ob/ob) mouse in reduced binding of purine nucleotides and a failure to respond to cold by an increase in binding. Biochem. Biophys. Res. Commun. 83, 628-634, 1978.

James, W. P. T. & Trayhurn, P.: Thermogenesis and obesity. Br. Med. Bull. 37, 43-48, 1981.

Johnson, M. L., Burke, B. S. & Mayer, J.: Relative importance of inactivity and overeating in the energy balance of obese high school girls. Am. J. Clin. Nutr. 4, 37-44, 1956.

Jung, R. T., Shetty, P. S., James, W. P. T., Barrard, M. & Callingham, B. A.: Reduced thermogenesis in obesity. Nature 279, 322-323, 1979.

Kleiber, M.: Dietary deficiencies and energy metabolism. Nutr. Abst. Rev. 15, 207-222, 1945.

McCracken, K. J. & Gray, R.: A futile energy cycle in adult rats given a low protein diet at high levels of energy intake. Proc. Nutr. Soc. 35, 59A-60A, 1976.

Miller, B. G., Otto, W. R., Grimble, R. F., York, D. A. & Taylor, T. G.: The relationship between protein turnover and energy balance in lean and genetically obese (ob/ob) mice. Br. J. Nutr. 42, 185-199, 1979.

Nicholls, D. G.: Brown adipose tissue mitochondria. Biochem. Biophys. Acta 549, 1-29, 1979.

Payne, P. R., and Dugdale, A. E.: A model for the prediction of energy balance and body weight. Ann. Human Biol., 4:525-535, 1962.

Perkins, M. N., Rothwell, N. J., Stock, M. J. & Stone, T. W.: Activation of brown adipose tissue thermogenesis by electrical stimulation of the ventromedial hypothalamus. J. Physiol. in press, 1980.

Pittet, Ph., Chappuis, Ph., Acheson, K., de Techtermann, F. & Jequier, E.: Thermic effect of glucose in obese subjects studied by direct and indirect calorimetry. Br. J. Nutr. 35, 281-292, 1976.

Rose, H. E. & Mayer, J.: Activity, caloric intake, fat storage, and the energy balance of infants. Pediatrics 41, 18-29, 1968.

Rothwell, N. J. & Stock, M. J.: A role for brown adipose tissue in diet- induced thermogenesis. Nature 281, 31-35, 1979.

Rothwell, N. J. & Stock, M. J.: A paradox in the control of energy intake in the rat. Nature 273, 146-147, 1978.

Rothwell, N. J. & Stock, M. J.: Regulation of energy balance in two models of reversible obesity in the rat. J. Comp. Physiol. Psychol. 93, 1024-1034, 1979.

Schutz, Y., Ravussin, E., Diethelm, R. & Jequier, E.: Spontaneous physical activity measured by radar in moderately obese and control subjects studies in a respiration chamber. Int. J. Obesity (In press), 1981.

Sims, E. A. H.: Experimental obesity, dietary-induced thermogenesis and their clinical implications. Clins Endocr. Metab. 5, 377-395, 1976.

Smith, R. E. & Horwitz, B. A.: Brown fat and thermogenesis. Physiol. Rev. 49, 330-425, 1969.

Stunkard, A. J. & Pestka, J.: The physical activity of obese girls. Am. J. Dis. Child. 103, 812, 1962.

Therriault, D. G., and Mellin, D. B.: Cellularity of adipose tissue in cold-exposed rats and the calorigenic effect of norepinephrine. Lipids, 6:486-491, 1971.

Thurlby, P. L. & Trayhurn, P.: The role of thermoregulatory thermogenesis in the development of obesity in genetically obese (ob/ob) mice pair fed with lean siblings. Br. J. Nutr. 42, 377-385, 1979.

Thurlby, P. L. & Trayhurn, P.: The role of environmental temperature in the excess energy gain of obese (ob/ob) mice pair fed to lean siblings. Br. J. Nutr. 42, 377-384, 1979.

Thurlby, P. L.: Studies on thermoregulatory thermogenesis in relation to energy balance in genetically obese (ob/ob) mice. Ph D Thesis, University of Cambridge, 1979.

Thurlby, P. L. & Trayhurn, P.: Regional blood flow in genetically obese (ob/ob) mice: the importance of brown adipose tissue to the reduced energy expenditure of non-shivering thermogenesis. Pflugers Arch. 385, 193-201, 1980.

Trayhurn, P. & James, W. P. T.: Thermoregulation and non-shivering thermogenesis in the genetically obese (ob/ob) mouse. Pflugers Arch. 373, 189-193, 1980.

Trayhurn, P., Thurlby, P. L., Woodward, C. J. H. & James, W. P. T.: Thermoregulation in genetically obese rodents: the relationship to metabolic efficiency. In Animal models of obesity, ed N. F. W. Festing, pp. 191-203. Macmillan, London, 1979.

Trayhurn, P., Thurlby, P. L., Goodbody, A. E. & James, W. P. T.: Brown adipose tissue and thermogenesis in obesity. In Proc. Serono Symp. in press, 1981.

Tulp, O., Frink, R., Sims, E. A. H. & Danforth, E.: Overnutrition induces hyperplasia of brown fat and diet-induced thermogenesis in the rat. Clin. Res. 28, 621A, 1980.

York, D. A., Morgan, J. B. & Taylor, T. G.: The relationship of dietary induced thermogenesis to metabolic efficiency in man. Proc. Nutr. Soc. 39, 57A, 1980.

Metabolic Factors

Allen, F. M.: The role of fat in diabetes. Am. J. Med. Sci. 153, 360-373, 1917.

Archer, J. A., Gorden, P. & Roth, J.: Defect in insulin binding to receptors in obese man. Amelioration with caloric restriction. J. Clin. Invest. 55, 166-174, 1975.

Assimacopoulos-Jeannet, F. & Jeanrenaud, B.: The hormonal and metabolic basis of experimental obesity. In Clinics in endocrinology and metabolism, Vol. 5, ed M. J. Albrink, pp. 337, 365. Saunders, Philadelphia, 1976.

Bar, R. S., Gordron, P., Roth, J., Kahn, C. R. & DeMeyts, P.: Fluctuations in the affinity and concentration of insulin receptors on circulating monocytes of obese patients: effects of starvation, refeeding and dieting. J. Clin. Invest. 58, 1123-1135, 1976.

Berger, M., Muller, W. A. & Renold, A. E.: Relationship of obesity to diabetes; some facts, many questions. In Advances in modern nutrition. II, ed H. M. Katzen & R. J. Mahler, pp. 211-228. Hemisphere Publ. Corp., 1977.

Bergstrom, J. & Hultman, E.: A study of the glycogen metabolism in man. J. Clin. Lab. Invest. 19, 218-229, 1967.

Bjorntorp, P., Fahlen, M., Grimsby, G., Gustafson, A., Holm, J., Renstrom, P. and Schersten, T.: Carbohydrate and lipid metabolism in middle-aged, physically well-trained men. Metabolism 21, 1037-1044, 1972.

Brunzell, J. D., Lerner, R. L., Hazzard, W. R., Porte, D. Jr. & Bierman, E. L.: Improved glucose tolerance with high carbohydrate feeding in mild diabetes. New Engl. J. Med. 284, 521-524, 1971.

Cherrington, A. D., Lacy, W. W. & Chaisson, J. L.: Effect of glucagon on glucose production during insulin deficiency in the dog. J. Clin. Invest. 62, 664-677, 1978.

Chiasson, J. L., Liljenquist, J. E., Lacy, W. W., Jennings, A. S. & Cherrington, A. D.: Gluconeogenesis: methodological approaches in vivo. Fed Proc. 36, 229-235, 1977.

Crettaz, M., Prentki, M., Zaninetti, D. & Jeanrenaud, B.: Insulin resistance in soleus muscle from obese Zucker rats. Involvement of several defective sites. Biochem. J. 186, 525-534, 1980.

Crofford, O. B. & Renold, A. E.: Glucose uptake by incubated rat epididymal adipose tissue. Characteristics of the glucose transport system and action of insulin. J. Biol. Chem. 240, 3237-3244, 1965.

Cuendet, G. S., Loten, E. G., Jeanrenaud, B. & Renold, A. E.: Decreased basal, non-insulin stimulated glucose uptake and metabolism by skeletal soleus muscle isolated from obese-hyperglycemic (ob/ob) mice. J. Clin. Invest. 58, 1078-1088, 1976.

Cushman, S. W. & Wardzala, L. J.: Potential mechanism of insulin action on glucose transport in the isolated rat adipose cell. Apparent translocation of intracellular transport systems to the plasma membrane. J. Biol. Chem. 255, 4758-4762, 1980.

Czech, M. P., Richardson, D. K. & Smith, C. J.: Biochemical basis of fat cell insulin resistance in obese rodents and man. Metabolism 26, 1057-1978, 1977.

Czech, M. D.: Cellular basis of insulin insensitivity in large rat adipocytes. J. Clin.Invest. 57, 1523-1532, 1976.

DeFronzo, R. A., Ferrannini, E., Hendler, R., Wahren, J. & Felig, P.: Influence of hyperinsulinemia, hyperglycemia, and the route of glucose administration on splanchic glucose exchange. Proc. Natl. Acad. Sci. 75, 5173-5177, 1978.

DiGirolamo, M. & Rudman, D.: Variations in glucose metabolism and sensitivity to insulin of the rat's adipose tissue, in relation to age and body weight. Endocrinology 82, 1133-1141, 1968.

Faber, O. K., Kehlet, H. & Christensen, K.: Hepatic insulin extraction in normal and obese man. 10th Cong. Int. Diabetes Fed. Vienna, 1979.

Faust, I. M. Johnson, P. R., Stern, J. S., et al.: Diet-induced adipocyte number increase in adult rats: a new model of obesity. Amer. J. Physiol., 235: E279-E286, 1978.

Felig, P. & Wahren, J.: The liver as site of insulin and glucagon action in normal, diabetic and obese humans. Ir. J. Med. Sci. 11, 528-539.

Gliemann, J., Gammeltoft, S. & Vinten, J.: Time course of insulin-receptor binding and insulin-induced lipogenesis in isolated rat fat cells. J. Biol. Chem. 250, 3368-3374, 1975.

Goldrick, R. B., and McLoughlin, G. M.: Lipolysis and lipogenesis from glucose in human fat cells of different sizes. Effects of insulin, epinephrine and theophylline. J. Clin. Invest., 49:1213-1223, 1970.

Insel, P. A., Liljenquist, J. E., Tobin, J. D., Sherwin, R. S., Watkins, P., Andres, R. & Berman, M.: Insulin control of glucose metabolism in man. J. Clin. Invest. 55, 1057-1066, 1975.

Issekutz, B.: Clearance rates of metabolizable and nonmetabolizable sugars in insulin-infused dogs and in exercising dogs. Diabetes 29, 348-354, 1980.

James, W. P. T. & Trayhurn, P.: An integrated view of the metabolic and genetic basis for obesity. Lancet 2, 770-773, 1976.

Jeanrenaud, B.: Adipose tissue dynamics and regulation, revisited. Ergebn. Physiol. 60, 57-141, 1968.

Jeanrenaud, B.: Insulin and obesity. Diabetologia 17, 133-138, 1919.

Johnson, P. R., Stern, J., Gruen, R., et al.: Development of adipose depot cellularity, plasma insulin, pancreatic insulin release and insulin resistance in the Zucker obese female rat. Fed. Proc., 35:657, 1976.

Kahn, C. R.: Role of insulin receptors in insulin-resistant states. Metabolism 29, 455-466, 1980.

Kahn, C. R., Neville, D. M., Jr. & Roth, J.: Insulin-receptor interaction in the obese hyperglycemic mouse. A model of insulin resistance. J. Biol. Chem. 248, 244-250, 1973.

Kalkhoff, R. K., Kim, H. J., Cerletty, J. et al.: Metabolic effects of weight loss in obese subjects: changes in plasma substrate levels, insulin and growth hormone responses. Diabetes 20, 83-91, 1971.

Karam, J. H., Grodsky, G. M. & Forsham, P. H.: Excessive insulin response to glucose in obese subjects as measured by immunochemical assay. Diabetes 12, 169-204, 1963.

Kolterman, O. G., Reaven, G. M. & Olefsky, J. M.: Relationship between in vivo insulin resistance and decreased insulin receptors in obese man. J. Clin. Endocr. Metab. 48, 487-494, 1979.

Kolterman, O. G., Insel, J., Saekow, M. & Olefsky, J. M.: Mechanisms of insulin resistance in human obesity: evidence for receptor and post-receptor defects. J. Clin. Invest. 65, 1272-1284, 1980.

Kono, T. & Barnham, F. W.: The relationship between the insulin-binding capacity of fat cells and the cellular response to insulin: studies with intact and trypsin-treated fat cells. J. Biol. Chem. 246, 6210-6216, 1971.

Kriesberg, R. A., Boshell, B. R., Di Placido, J. & Roddam, R. F.: Insulin secretion in obesity. New Engl. J. Med. 276, 314-319, 1976.

Krotkiewski, M., Sjostrom, L., Bjorntorp, P., Carlgren, G., Garellick, C. & Smith, U.: Adipose tissue cellularity in relation to prognosis for weight reduction. Int. J. Obesity 1, 395-416, 1977.

LeMarchand-Brustel, Y., Jean-Renaud, B. & Freychet, P.: Insulin binding and effects in isolated soleus muscle of lean and obese mice. Am. J. Physiol. 234, E348-E358, 1978.

LeMarchand, Y., Freychet, P. & Jeanrenaud, B.: Longitudinal study on the establishment of insulin resistance in hypothalamic obese mice. Endocrinology 102, 74-85, 1978.

Levine, R. & Goldstein, M.: On the mechanism of action of insulin. Recent Prog. Horm. Res. 11, 343-380, 1955.

Livingston, J. N. & Lockwood, D. H.: Direct measurement of sugar uptake in small and large adipocytes from young and adult rats. Biochem. Biophys. Res. Commun. 61, 989-996, 1974.

Ogilvie, R. F.: Sugar tolerance in obese subjects. A review by 64 cases. Quart. J. Med. 4, 345-358, 1935.

Ogilvie, R. F.: The islands of Langerhans in 19 cases of obesity. J. Pathol. Bacteriol. 37, 473-481, 1933.

Olefsky, J. M., Reaven, G. M. & Farquhar, J. W.: Effects of weight reduction on obesity: studies of carbohydrate and lipid metabolism. J. Clin. Invest. 53, 64-76, 1974.

Olefsky, J. M.: The insulin receptor: its role in insulin resistance of obesity and diabetes. Diabetes 25, 1154-1165, 1976.

Olefsky, J. M.: The effects of spontaneous obesity on insulin binding, glucose transport and glucose oxidation of isolated rat adipocytes. J. Clin. Invest. 57, 842-851, 1976.

Olefsky, J. M.: Decreased insulin binding to adipocytes and circulating monocytes from obese subjects. J. Clin. Invest. 57, 1165-1177, 1976.

Poggi, C., LeMarchand-Brustel, Y., Zapf, J., Froesch, E. R. & Freychet, P.: Effects and binding of insulin-like growth factor I in the isolated soleus muscle of lean and obese mice: Comparison with insulin. Endocrinology 105, 723-730, 1979.

Rabinowitz, D.: Some endocrine and metabolic aspects of obesity. Ann. Rev. Med. 21, 241-258, 1970.

Rabinowitz, D. & Zierler, K. L.: Forearm metabolism in obesity and its response to intra-arterial insulin. J. Clin. Invest. 41, 2173-2181, 1962.

Reaven, G. M. & Olefsky, J. M.: Role of insulin resistance in the pathogenesis of hyperglycemia. In Advances in modern nutrition, 2, pp. 229-266, J. Willey and Sons, London, 1978.

Reiser, S., and Hallfrisch, J.: Insulin sensitivity and adipose tissue weight of rats fed starch or sucrose diets ad libitum or in meals. J. Nutr., 107:147-155, 1977.

Reiser, S., Hallfrisch, J., Putney, J., et al.: Enhancement of intestinal sugar transport by rats fed sucrose as compared to starch. Nutr. Metab., 20:461-470, 1976.

Salans, L. B., Knittle, J. L. & Hirsch, J.: The role of adipose cell size and adipose tissue insulin sensitivity in the carbohydrate intolerance of human obesity. J. Clin. Invest. 47, 153, 1968.

Salans, L. B., Bray, G. A., Cushman, S. W., Danforth, E. Jr., Glennon, J. A., Horton, E. S. & Sims, E. A. H.: Glucose metabolism and the response to insulin by human adipose tissue in spontaneous and experimental obesity. Effects of dietary composition and adipose cell size. J. Clin. Invest, 53, 848, 1974.

Salans, L. B. & Cushman, S. W.: Relationship of adiposity and diet to the abnormalities of carbohydrate metabolism in obesity. In Diabetes, obesity and vascular disease. Advances in modern nutrition, vol. 2., ed H. M. Hatzen & R. J. Mahler. Wiley and Sons, New York, 1978.

Salans, L. B. & Dougherty, J. W.: The effect of insulin upon glucose metabolism by adipose cells of difficult size. Influence of cell lipid and protein content, age, and nutritional state. J. Clin. Invest. 50, 1399-1410, 1971.

Schteingart, D. E., Gregerman, R. I. & Conn, J. W.: A comparison of the characteristics of increased adrenocorticol function in obesity and in Cushing's syndrome. Metabolism 12, 484-497, 1963.

Schwartz, R. S. & Brunzell, J. D.: Possible role of adipose tissue lipo- protein lipase in the maintenance of obesity in man. Clin. Res. 28, 82, 1980.

Seidman, I., Horland, A. A. & Teebor, G. W.: Glycolytic and gluconeogenic enzyme activities in the hereditary obese-hyperglycemic syndrome and in acquired obesity. Diabetologia 6, 313-316, 1970.

Sims, E. A. H., Danforth, E. Jr., Horton, E. S., Bray, G. A., Glennon, J. A. & Salans, L. B.: Endocrine and metabolic effects of experimental obesity in man. Recent Prog. Horm. Res. 29, 457-476, 1973.

Sjostrom, L., Garellick, G., Krotkiewski, M. & Luyckx, A.: Peripheral insulin in response to the sight and smell of food. Metabolism 29, 901-9, 1980.

Soll, A. H., Kahn, C. R. & Neville, D. M., Jr.: Insulin binding to liver plasma membranes in the obese hyperglycemic (ob/ob) mouse. Demonstration of a decreased number of functionally normal receptors. J. Biol. Chem. 250, 4702-4707, 1975.

Soll, A. H., Kahn, C. R., Neville, D. M., Jr., et al.: Insulin receptor deficiency in genetic and acquired obesity. J. Clin. Invest., 56:769, 1975.

Steffens, A. B.: Influence of reversible obesity on eating behavior, blood glucose and insulin in the rat. Amer. J. Physiol. 208:1-5, 1975.

Stern, M., Olefsky, J., Farquhar, J., et al.: Relationship between fat cell size and insulin resistance in vivo. Clin. Res. 20:557, 1972.

Van Itallie, T. B.: Dietary fiber and obesity. Amer. J. Clin. Nutr., 31: S43-S52, 1978.

Wardzala, L. J., Cushman, S. W. & Salans, L. B.: Mechanism of insulin action on glucose transport in the isolated rat adipose cell. Enhancement of the number of functional transport systems. J. Biol. Chem. 253, 8002-8005, 1978.

Yalow, R. S., Glick, S. M., Roth, J. & Berson, S. A.: Plasma insulin and growth hormone levels in obesity and diabetes. Ann. N. Y. Acad. Sci. 131, 357-373, 1965.

York, D. A., Steinke, J. & Bray, G. A.: Hyperinsulinemia and insulin resistance in genetically obese rats. Metabolism 21, 277-284, 1972.

Obesity and Exercise

Askew, E. W., Huston, R. L., Plopper, C. G. & Hecker, A. L.: Adipose tissue cellularity and lipolysis. Response to exercise and cortisol treatment. J. Clin. Invest. 56, 521-529, 1975.

Bar-Or, O., Lundergren, H. M. & Burskirk, E. R.: Heat tolerance of exercising obese and lean women. J. Appl. Physiol. 26, 403-409, 1969.

Berchtold, P., Berger, M., Finke, C. & Burger, A.: Hormonelle Veranderungen wahrend des Fastens. Schweiz. Med. Wschr. 110, 966-968, 1980.

Berger, M., Berchtold, P. & Kemmer, F. W.: Diabetes and exercise. In Handbook of diabetes mellitis, III, ed M. Brownlee, pp. 273-305. Garland Press, New York, 1980.

Berger, M., Kemmer, F. W., Becker, K., Herberg, L., Schwenen, M., Gjinavci, A. & Berchtold, P.: Effects of physical training on glucose tolerance and on glucose metabolism of skeletal muscle in anaesthetized normal rats. Diabetologia 16, 179-184, 1979.

Bjorntorp, P.: Exercise in the treatment of obesity. In Clins. Endocr. Metab. ed M. J. Albrink, pp. 431-453. Saunders, London, 1976.

Bjorntorp, P., de Jounge, K., Sjostrom, L. and Sullivan, L.: Physical training in human obesity. II. Effects on plasma insulin in glucose-intolerant subjects without marked hyperinsulinemia. Scandinavian Journal of Clinical and Laboratory Investigation 32, 41, 1973.

Bjorntorp, P., de Jounge, K., Krotkiewski, M., Sullivan, L., Sjostrom, L. and Stenberg, J.: Physical training in human obesity. III. Effects of long-term physical training on body composition. Metabolism 22, 1467, 1973.

Bjorntorp, P., de Jounge, K., Sjostrom, L. and Sullivan, L.: The effect of physical training on insulin production in obesity. Metabolism 19, 631, 1970.

Bjorntorp, P., Berchtold, P., Grimby, G., Lindholm, B., Sanne, H., Tibblin, G. and Wilhelmsen, L.: Effects of physical training on glucose tolerance, plasma insulin and lipids and on body composition in men after myocardial infarction. Acta Medica Scandinavica 192:439, 1972.

Bjorntorp, P., de Jounge, K., Krotkiewski, M., Sullivan, L., Sjostrom, L. & Sternberg, J.: Physical training in human obesity. III. Effects of long-term physical training on body composition. Metabolism 22, 1467-1475, 1973.

Bjorntorp, P., Holm, G., Jacobsson, B., Schiller-de Jounge, K., Lundberg, P-A., Sjbstrom, L., Smith, U. & Sullivan, L.: Physical training in human hyperplastic obesity. IV. Effects of the hormonal status. Metabolism 26, 319-327, 1977.

Bjorntorp, P.: Effects of physical conditioning in obesity. In Obesity in perspective, ed G. A. Bray, pp. 397-406. DHEW-Publication (NIH) 75:708. Bethesda, Maryland, USA, 1975.

Bogardus, C., Danforth, E. Jr., LaGrange, B. M., Horton, E. S. & Sims, E. A. H.: Metabolic effects of hypocaloric diets with or without carbohydrate and the capacity for exercise. Clin. Res. 28, 646A, 1980.

Bradfield, R. & Curtis, D.: Effect of activity on caloric response of obese women. Am. J. Clin. Nutr. 21, 1208-1210, 1968.

Bray, G. A., Whipp, B. J., Koyal, S. N. & Wasserman, K.: Some respiratory and metabolic effects of exercise in moderately obese men. Metabolism 26, 403-412, 1977.

Buskirk, E. R.. Thompson, R. H., Lutwak, L. & Whedon, G. D.: Energy Balance of obese patients during weight reduction: influence of diet restriction and exercise. Ann. N.Y. Acad. Sci. 110, 918-940, 1963.

Buskirk, E. R.: Obesity: a brief overview with emphasis on exercise. Fed. Proc. 33, 1948-1951, 1974.

Costill, D. L., Jansson, E., Golnick, P. D. & Saltin, B.: Glycogen utilization in leg muscles of men during level and uphill running. Acta Physiol. Scand. 91, 475-481, 1974.

Cuppers, H. J., Erdmann, R., Schubert, H., Berchtold, P. & Berger, M.: Glucose tolerance, serum insulin, and serum lipids in athletes. Int. Symp. "Diabetes and exercise", Olympia, Greece, 1980.

Dempsey, J. A., Redden, W., Balke, B. & Rankin, J.: Work capacity determinants and physiological cost of weight supported work in obesity. J. Appl. Physiol. 21, 1815-1820, 1966.

Dempsey, J.: Exercise and obesity. In Sports medicine, ed A. J. Ryan & F. L. Allman, Jr., pp. 557-593. Academic Press, New York, 1974.

Dudleston, A. K. & Bennion, M.: Effect of diet and/or exercise on obese college women. J. Am. Med. Ass. 56, 126-129, 1970.

Durnin, J. V. G. A.: Possible interaction between physical activity, body composition and obesity in man. In Recent advances in obesity research, II, ed G. A. Bray, pp. 237-241. Newman, London, 1978.

Editorial: Successful diet and exercise therapy is conducted in Vermont for "Diabesity". J. Am. Med. Ass. 243, 519-520, 1980.

Epstein, Leonard, and Wing, Rena: Aerobic Exercise and Weight, Addictive Behaviors 5, 371-88(1980). Erratum, ibid. 6, 183, 1981.

Fahlen, M., Stenberg, J. & Bjorntorp, P.: Insulin secretion in obesity after exercise. Diabetologia 8, 141-144, 1972.

Felig, P. & Wahren, J.: Fuel homeostasis in exercise. New Engl. J. Med. 293, 1078-1084, 1975.

Foss, M. L., Lampman, R. M., Watt, E. & Schteingart, D. E.: Initial work tolerance of extremely obese patients. Archs Phys. Med. Rehabil. 56, 63-67, 1975.

Foss, M. L., Lampman, R. M. & Schteingart, D. E.: Physical training program for rehabilitating extremely obese patients. Archs Phys. Med. Rehabil. 57, 425-429, 1976.

Foss, M. L., Lampman, R. M. & Schteingart, D. E.: Extremely obese patients: improvements in exercise tolerance with physical training and weight loss. Archs Phys. Med. Rehabil. 61, 119-124, 1980.

Franklin, B., Buskirk, E., Hodgson, J., Gahagan, H., Kollias, J. & Mendez, J.: Effects of physical conditioning on cardio-respiratory function, body composition and serum lipids in relatively normal-weight and obese middle-aged women. Int. J. Obesity 3, 97-109, 1979.

Galbo, H., Holst, J. J. & Christensen, N. J.: The effect of different diets and of insulin on the hormonal response to prolonged exercise. Acta Physiol. Scand. 107, 19-32, 1979.

Galbo, H., Hedeskov, C. J. & Capito, K.: Effect of physical training on insulin secretion of rat pancreatic islets. 10th Congr. Int. Diabetes Fed. Vienna, 1979.

Gonzalez, Elizabeth Rasche: Exercise Therapy "Rediscovered" for Diabetes, But What Does It Do? Journal of the Amer. Med. Assoc. 242, 1591-92, 1979.

Gordon, R., Spector, S., Sjoerdsma, A. & Undenfriend, S.: Increased synthesis of norepinephrine and epinephrine in the intact rat during exercise and exposure to cold. J. Pharmac. Exp. Ther. 153, 440-447, 1966.

Gwinup, G.: Effect of exercise alone on weight of obese women. Archs Intern. Med. 135, 676-680, 1975.

Gyntelberg, F., Brennan, R., Holloszy, J. O., Schonfeld, G., Rennie, M. J. & Weidman, S. W.: Plasma triglyceride lowering by exercise despite increased food intake in patients with type IV hyperlipoproteinemia. Am. J. Clin. Nutr. 30, 716-720, 1977.

Harger, B. S., Miller, J. B. & Thomas, J. C.: The caloric cost of running. Its impact on weight reduction. J. Am. Med. Ass. 228, 482-483, 1974.

Hartley, L. H., Mason, J. W., Hogan, R. P., Jones, L. G., Kotchen, T. A., Mougey, E. H., Wherry, F. E., Pennington, L. L. & Ricketts, P. T.: Multiple hormonal responses to graded exercise in relation to physical training. J. Appl. Physiol. 33, 602-606, 1972.

Havel, R. J., Pernow, B. & Jones, J. L.: Uptake and release of free fatty acids and other metabolites in legs of exercising men. J. Appl. Physiol. 23, 90-96, 1976.

Holm, G. Bjorntorp, P. & Jagenburg, R.: Effects on carbohydrate, lipid and amino acid metabolism during the days following a submaximal physical exercise in man. J. Appl. Physiol. 45, 128-131, 1978.

Hultman, E.: Studies on muscle metabolism of glycogen and active phosphate in man with special reference to exercise and diet. Scand. J. Clin. Lab. Invest. 19(Suppl.94), 1-63, 1967.

Hursh, L. M.: Exercise in weight reduction. Nebraska Med. J. 61, 158-160, 1976.

Huttunen, J. K., Lansimies, E., Voutilainen, E., Ehnholm, C., Hietanen, E., Penttila, I., Slitonen, O. & Rauramaa, R.: Effect of moderate physical exercise on serum lipoproteins. A controlled clinical trial with special reference to serum high-density lipoproteins. Circulation 60, 1220-1229, 1979.

Kenrick, M. M., Ball, M. F. & Canary, J. J.: Exercise and weight reduction in obesity. Archs Phsy. Med. Rehabil. 63, 323-327, 340, 1972.

Koivisto, V. A., Soman, V., Conrad, P., Hendler, R., Nadel, E. & Felig, P.: Insulin binding to monocytes in trained athletes. Changes in the resting state and after exercise. J. Clin. Invest. 64, 1011-1015, 1979.

Koivisto, V. A., Soman, V. R. & Felig, P.: Effects of acute exercise on insulin binding to monocytes in obesity. Metabolism 29, 168-171, 1980.

Krotkiewski, M., Sjostrom, L., and Sullivan, L.: Effects of long-term training on adipose tissue cellularity and body composition in hypertrophic and hyperplastic obesity. Internat. J. Obesity, 2:395, 1977.

Krotkiewski, M., Sjostrom, L. & Bjorntorp, P.: Physical training in hyperplastic obesity. V. Effects of atropine on plasma insulin. Int. J. Obesity 4, 49-56, 1980.

LeBlanc, J., Nadeau, A., Boulay, M. & Rousseau-Migneron, S.: Effects of physical training and adiposity on glucose metabolism and 'I-insulin binding. J. Appl. Physiol. 235-239, 1979.

Leon, Arthur, et al.: Effects of a Vigorous Walking Program on Body Composition, and Carbohydrate and Lipid Metabolism of Obese Young Men, American Journal of Clinical Nutrition 32, 1776-87, 1979.

Lewis, S., Haskell, W. L., Wood, P. D., Manoogian, N., Bailey, J. E. & Pereira, M. B.: Effects of physical activity on weight reduction in obese middle-aged women. Am. J. Clin. Nutr. 29, 151-156, 1976.

Lithell, H., Hellsing, K., Lundqvist, G. & Malmberg, P.: Lipoprotein-lipase activity of human skeletal-muscle and adipose tissue after intensive physical exercise. Acta Physiol. Scand. 105, 312-315, 1979.

Lohmann, D., Liebold, F., Heilmann, W., Seuger, H. and Pohl, A.: Diminished insulin response in highly trained athletes. Metabolism 27, 521, 1978.

Maehlum, S. & Pruett, E. D.: Muscular exercise and metabolism in male juvenile diabetics. II. Glucose tolerance after exercise. Scand. J. Clin. Lab. Invest. 32, 149-153, 1973.

Maehlum, S., Felig, P. & Wahren, J.: Splanchnic glucose and muscle glycogen metabolism after glucose feeding during post exercise recovery. Am. J. Physiol. 235, E255-E260, 1978.

Mayer, J.: Exercise and weight control. In Science and medicine of exercise and sport, ed W. Johnson, Harper, New York, 1960.

Mayer J., Marshall, N. B., Vitale, J. J., Christensen, J. H., Mashayckhi,- M. B. & Stare, F. J.: Exercise, food intake and body weight in normal rats and genetically obese mice. Am. J. Physiol. 177, 544-548, 1954.

Mondon, C. E. & Dolkas, C. D.: Enhanced glucose uptake and insulin sensitivity in skeletal muscle from exercise-trained rats at rest. Diabetes 28, 381, 1979.

Moody, D. L., Kollias, J., and Buskirk, E. R.: The Effect of a Moderate Exercise Program on Body Weight and Skinfold Thickness in Overweight College Women, Medicine and Science in Sports 1(no. 2, 75-80, 1969.

Nikkila, E., Taskinen, M. R., Rehunen, S. & Harkonen, M.: Lipoprotein lipase activity in adipose tissue and skeletal muscle of runners: relation to serum lipoproteins. Metabolism 27, 1661-1671, 1978.

Oscai, L. B. & Holloszy, J. O.: Effects of weight changes produced by exercise, food restriction, or overeating on body composition. J. Clin. Invest. 48, 2124-2128, 1969.

Oscai, L. B., Patterson, J. A., Bogard, D. L., Beck, R. J. & Rothermel, B. L.: Normalization of serum triglycerides and lipoprotein electrophoretic patterns by exercise. Am. J. Cardiol. 30, 775-780, 1972.

Oscai, L. B.: The role of exercise in weight control. In Exercise and sports reviews. I. pp. 103-123, Academic Press, London, 1973.

Owens, J. L., Fuller, E. O., Nutter, D. O. & DiGirolamo, M.: Influence of moderate exercise on adipocyte metabolism and hormonal responsiveness. J. Appl. Physiol. 43, 425-430, 1977.

Parizkova, J. & Stankova, L.: Influence of physical activity on a treadmill on the metabolism of adipose tissue in rats. Br. J. Nutr. 18, 325-332, 1964.

Parizkova, J.: Impact of age, diet and exercise on man's body composition. Ann. N.Y. Acad. Sci. 110, 661-674, 1963.

Parizkova, J.: Body fat and physical fitness. 209-222, 252-261. The Hague: M. Nijhoff, 1977.

Pedersen, Oluf, Beck-Nielsen, Henning, & Heding, Lise: Increased Insulin Receptors After Exercise in Patients with Insulin-Dependent Diabetes Mellitus, New England Journal of Medicine 302, 886-92, 1980.

Phinney, S. D., Horton, E. S., Sims, E. A. H., Hanson, J. S., Danforth, E. J. & LaGrange, B. M.: Capacity for moderate exercise in obese subjects after adaptation to a hypocaloric, ketogenic diet. J. Clin. Invest. 66, 1152-1160, 1980.

Pollock, M. L., Miller, H. S. Jr., Linnerud, A. C., Robertson, B. & Valentino, R.: Effects of walking on body composition and cardiovascular function of middle-aged men. J. Appl. Physiol. 30, 126-130, 1971.

Pruett, E. D. R.: Fat and carbohydrate metabolism in exercise and recovery, and its dependence upon work load severity. Academic Dissertation, Institute of Work Physiology, University of Oslo, 1971.

Ruderman, N. B., Ganda, O. P., Johansen, K.: The effect of physical training on glucose tolerance and plasma lipids in maturity-onset diabetes. Diabetes 28, suppl. 1, 89-92, 1979.

Saltin, B., Lindgarde, F., Lithell, H., Eriksson, K. F. & Gad, P.: Metabolic effects of long-term physical training in maturity onset diabetes. In Diabetes 1979, ed W. K. Waldhausl, pp. 345-350. Amsterdam: Excerpta Medica, 1980.

Schteingart, D. E., Foss, M. L., Lampman, R. M., Short, M., Buntman, H., Michael, R. & McGowan, J.: Obesity - a multidisciplinary approach to management. In Recent advances in obesity research, I ed A. Howard, pp. 304-307. Newman, London, 1975.

Maja Schade et al.: Spot Reducing in Overweight College Women, Research Quarterly 33; 461-71, 1962.

Sidney, K. H., Shephard, R. J. & Harrison, J. E.: Endurance training and body composition of the elderly. Am. J. Clin. Nutr. 30, 326-333, 1977.

Soman, V. R., Koivisto, V. A., Deibert, D., Felig, P. & DeFronzo, R. A.: Increased insulin sensitivity and insulin binding to monocytes after physical training. New Engl. J. Med. 301, 1200-1204, 1979.

Soman, V. R., Koivisto, V. A., Grantham, P. & Felig, P.: Increased insulin binding to monocytes after acute exercise in normal man. J. Clin. Endocr. Metab. 47, 216-219, 1978.

Sullivan, L.: Metabolic and physiologic effects of physical training in hyperplastic obesity. Scand. J. Rehabil. Med. Suppl. 5, 1-38, 1976.

Turell, E. T., Austin, R. C. & Alexander, J. K.: Cardio-respiratory responses of very obese subjects to treadmill exercise. J. Lab. Clin. Invest. 64, 107, 1964.

Vranic, M. & Berger, M.: Exercise and diabetes mellitus. Diabetes 28, 147-167, 1979.

Wardzala, L., Horton, E., Horton, E., Jeanrenaud, B.: Physical training increases glucose transport and metabolism in rat adipose cells without altering insulin binding or sensitivity. Proc. 3rd Int. Cong. Obesity (Rome 1980). Alim. Nutr. Metab. 1, 376 (Abstract), 1980.

Wells, B. J., Parizkova, J. & Jokl, E.: Exercise, excess fat and body weight. J. Ass. Phys. Ment. Rehab. 16, 35-40, 1962.

Weltman, A., Matter, S. & Stamford, B. A.: Caloric restriction and/or mild exercise: effects on serum lipids and body composition. Am. J. Clin. Nutr. 33, 1002-1009, 1980.

Wertz, S. H. & Wertz, R. L.: Exercise and diet as therapeutic aids in weight reduction and subsequent control. Am. Corr. Ther. J. 21, 122-130, 1976.

Wirth, A., Diehm, C. & Bjorntorp, P.: Plasma insulin and C-peptide during exercise in trained and untrained subjects. Int. Symp.'Diabetes and Exercise'. Olympia, Greece, 1980.

Wirth, A., Diehm, C., Mayer, H., Morl, H., Vogel, I., Bjorntorp, P. & Schlierf, G.: Plasma C-peptide and insulin in trained and untrained subjects. J. Appl. Physiol. in press, 1981.

Wirth, A., Holm, G., Nilsson, B., Smith, U. & Bjorntorp, P.: Insulin kinetics and insulin binding to adipocytes in physically trained and food-restricted rats. Am. J. Physiol. 238, E108-E115, 1980.

Wolf, L. M., Courtois, H., Javet, H. & Schrub, J. C.: Physical training associated with semi-starvation in the treatment of obesity. In Recent advances in obesity research, I, ed A. Howard, pp. 281-283, Newman, London, 1975.

Obesity and Diet

Bistrian, B. R., Blackburn, G. L., Flatt, J. P., et al.: Nitrogen metabolism and insulin requirements in obese adults on a protein-sparing modified fast. Diabetes, 25:494-504, 1975.

Bistrian, B. R.: Clinical use of the protein-sparing modified fast. J.A.M.A., 240:2299-2302, 1978.

Bjorntorp, P., Carlgren, G., Isaksson, B., Krotkiewski, M., Larsson, B. & Sjorstrom, L.: The effect of and energy reducing dietary regime in relation to adipose tissue cellularity in obese women. Am. J. Clin. Nutr. 28, 445, 1975.

Blackburn, G. L.: The liquid protein controversy: a closer look at the facts. Obesity Bariat. Med., 7:25-28, 1978.

Braunstein, J. J.: Management of the obese patient. Med. Clin. N. Am. 55, 391-401, 1971.

Bray, G. A.: Treatment of the obese patient: Use of diet and exercise. In The Obese Patient, W. B. Saunders Co., Philadelphia, 1976.

Bray, G. A.: Clinical management of the obese adult. Postgrad, Med, 51, 125-129, 1972.

Bray, G. A.: The myth of diet in the management of obesity. Am. J, Clin, Nutr. 23, 1141, 1970.

DeHaven, J., Sherwin, R., Hendler, R. & Felig, P. Nitrogen and sodium balance and sympathetic-nervous-system activity in obese subjects treated with a low-calorie protein or mixed diet. New Engl. J. Med, 302, 477-482, 1980,

Drenick, E. J. & Johnsson, D.: Weight reduction by fasting and semistarvation in morbid obesity: long-term follow-up. Int. J. Obesity 2, 123-132, 1978.

Garrow, J.: How to treat and when to treat. In The treatment of obesity, ed J. F. Munro, pp. 1-19. MTP Press Limited, Lancaster, 1979.

Goldberg, L., and Dornfeld, L.: Cardiac complications of liquid protein diets. J.A.M.A., 240:2542, 1978.

Isaksson, B.: Diet and Exercise. Assessment of the Swedish Program. In Bray, G., ed.: Recent Advances in Obesity Research: II., pp. 477-485, Newman, London, 1978.

Lindner, P. G., and Blackburn, G. L.: Multidisciplinary approach to obesity utilizing fasting modified by protein-sparing therapy. Obesity Bariat. Med., 5:198-216, 1976.

McClellan, W. S., Rupp, V. R. & Toscani, V.: Clinical calorimetry. XLVI. Prolonged meat diets with a study of the metabolism of nitrogen, calcium, and phosphorus. J. Biol. Chem. 87, 669-680, 1930.

MacCuish, A. C., Munro, J. F. & Duncan, L. J. P.: Follow up study of refractory obesity treated by fasting. Br. Med. J. 1, 91, 1968.

Parizkova, J., Vaneckova, M., Sprynarova, S. & Vamerova, M.: Body composition and fitness in obese children before and after special treatment. Acta

Paediat. Scand. Suppl. 217, 80, 1971. Sebrell, W. H.: The nutritional adequacy of Reducing Diets. In Howard, A., ed.: Recent Advances in Obesity Research: I. Proceedings of the 1st International Congress on Obesity, Newman Publishing, London, 1975.

Psychological Factors

Abramson, E. & Stinson, S. G.: The effects of boredom on eating. Addict. Behav. 2, 181-185, 1977.

Gates, J. C., Huenemann, R. L. & Brand, R. J.: Food choices of obese and non-obese persons. J. Am. Diet. Ass. 67, 339, 1975.

Herman, C. P. & Mack, D.: Restrained and unrestrained eating. J. Personality 43, 647-660, 1975.

McKenna, R. J.: Some effects of anxiety level and food cues in the behavior of obese and normal subjects. J. Personality Soc. Psychol. 221, 311-319, 1972.

Parent, E.A.: Anger and Weight Control: A Comparison of the Effects of Rational Anger Management versus Relaxation Training with Obese Females in conjunction with a Behavior Modification-Exercise Treatment Program, Dissertation, Brigham Young University, 1982. Provo, Utah.

Robbins, T. & Fray, P.: Stress-inducing eating: Fact, fiction or misunderstanding? Appetite 1, 103-133, 1980.

Robinson, S. & Winnik, H.: Psychotic disturbances following crash diet weight loss. Archs Gen. Psychol. 29, 559-562, 1973.

Schachter, S., Goldman, R. & Gordon, A.: Effects of fear, food deprivation, and obesity on eating. J. Personality Soc. Psychol. 10, 91-97, 1968.

Slochower, J.: Emotional labeling and overeating in obese and normal weight individuals. Psychosom. Med. 38, 131-139, 1976.

Spitzer, L., Marcus, J. & Rodin, J.: Arousal induced eating: A response to Robbins and Fray. Appetite, (in press).

Stuart, R. B., and Guire, K.: Some correlates of the maintenance of weight loss through behavior modification. Internat. J. Obes., 2:225-235, 1978.

Stunkard, A. J., and Penick, S.: Behavior modification in the treatment of obesity: The problem of maintaining weight loss. Arch. Gen. Psychiat., 36:801-806, 1979.

Stunkard, A. J.: Behavioral treatment of obesity: The current status. Internat. J. Obesity, 2:237-249, 1978.

Stunkard, A. J. & Penick, S. B.: Behavior modification in the treatment of obesity. The problem of maintaining weight loss. Archs Gen. Psychiatry 36, 801-806, 1979.

Wilson, G. T.: Behavior therapy and the treatment of obesity. In Addict. disorders. Pergamon Press, New York, 1980.

Wilson, G. T., and Brownell, K. D.: Behavior therapy for obesity: Including family members in the treatment process. Behav. Ther., 9:943-945, 1978.

Wooley, S. C., Wooley, O. W., and Dyrenforth, S. R.: Theoretical, practical, and social issues in behavioral treatments of obesity. J. Appl. Behav. Anal., 12:3-25, 1979.

Wooley, O. W., Wooley, S. C. & Dyrenforth, S.: Obesity and women, II: A neglected feminist topic. Women's Studies International Quarterly, (in press).

Wooley, O. W. & Wooley, S. C.: The experimental psychology of obesity. In Obesity: its pathogenesis and management. ed T. Silverstone & J. Finchman. Lancaster, England: Medical and Technical Publishing, 1975.

INDEX

Daily Record

Date _____

Day	Meal	Time	Amount	Item	RCU	FU	D U	H
Exercise				Water	Total			

Exercise				Water	Total			

Meal:**B** = breakfast, **L** = light meal, **M** = main meal, **S** = snack.
H = hunger. Put an X for no hunger prior to snack

End of Main Meal Hunger/Satiety	Points
Completely satisfied	10
No hunger, but not completely satisfied	8
Slightly overfull or mild hunger	5
Definately overfull or moderate hunger	0

Daily Record

Date _____

Day	Meal	Time	Amount	Item	RCU	FU	DU	H
Exercise				Water	Total			

Exercise				Water	Total			

Meal:**B** = breakfast, **L** = light meal, **M** = main meal, **S** = snack.
H = hunger. Put an X for no hunger prior to snack

End of Main Meal Hunger/Satiety	Points
Completely satisfied	10
No hunger, but not completely satisfied	8
Slightly overfull or mild hunger	5
Definately overfull or moderate hunger	0

Daily Record

Date _____

Day	Meal	Time	Amount	Item	RCU	FU	D U	H
Exercise				Water	Total			

Day	Meal	Time	Amount	Item	RCU	FU	D U	H
Exercise				Water	Total			

Meal: **B** = breakfast, **L** = light meal, **M** = main meal, **S** = snack.
H = hunger. Put an X for no hunger prior to snack

End of Main Meal Hunger/Satiety	Points
Completely satisfied	10
No hunger, but not completely satisfied	8
Slightly overfull or mild hunger	5
Definately overfull or moderate hunger	0

Daily Record

Date _____

Day	Meal	Time	Amount	Item	RCU	FU	D U	H
Exercise				Water	Total			
Exercise				Water	Total			

Meal: **B** = breakfast, **L** = light meal, **M** = main meal, **S** = snack.
H = hunger. Put an X for no hunger prior to snack

End of Main Meal Hunger/Satiety	**Points**
Completely satisfied	10
No hunger, but not completely satisfied	8
Slightly overfull or mild hunger	5
Definately overfull or moderate hunger	0

Daily Record

Date _____

Day	Meal	Time	Amount	Item	RCU	FU	D U	H
Exercise				Water	Total			
Exercise				Water	Total			

Meal: **B** = breakfast, **L** = light meal, **M** = main meal, **S** = snack.
H = hunger. Put an X for no hunger prior to snack

End of Main Meal Hunger/Satiety	Points
Completely satisfied	10
No hunger, but not completely satisfied	8
Slightly overfull or mild hunger	5
Definately overfull or moderate hunger	0

Daily Record

Date _____

Day	Meal	Time	Amount	Item	RCU	FU	DU	H
Exercise			Water		Total			

Day	Meal	Time	Amount	Item	RCU	FU	DU	H
Exercise			Water		Total			

Meal: **B** = breakfast, **L** = light meal, **M** = main meal, **S** = snack.
H = hunger. Put an X for no hunger prior to snack

End of Main Meal Hunger/Satiety	**Points**
Completely satisfied	10
No hunger, but not completely satisfied	8
Slightly overfull or mild hunger	5
Definately overfull or moderate hunger	0

Easy Gourmet Menus
To Lower Your Fat Thermostat

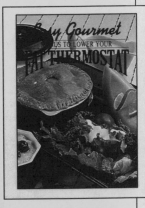

The latest from Chef Howard Gifford, author of *Gifford's Gourmet Delites*. Low-fat gourmet cooking made easy. The 32 menus with over 180 irresistible recipes (including those presented by Chef Gifford on the popular Midday Show on KSL television, Salt Lake City, Utah) makes *Easy Gourmet Menus* a must for your cookbook library. Each easy to follow recipe gives the option of using his new conveniently packaged spice mixes (see ad below) or your own individual spices. Either way you'll be delighted with the taste of these wonderfully delicious meals.

Gifford's Spice Mixes

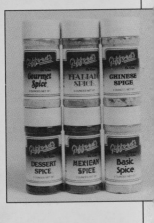

Chef Howard Gifford has just made your cooking easier. Now the unique flavors created by Chef Gifford can be had at the shake of a bottle. Eliminate the cupboard full of spices that are seldom used. Cut the time of mixing and measuring spices. No more guess-work to create a desired taste. These new spice mixes are conveniently packaged with six inviting flavors; Gourmet Spice, Mexican Spice, Basic Spice, Italian Spice, Chinese Spice, and Dessert Spice. Use these spice mixes with the delicious recipes in the new book *Easy Gourmet Menus to Lower Your Fat Thermostat* or flavor your own meals with desired spice mix. You'll be delighted at the results.

Gifford's Gourmet De-Lites

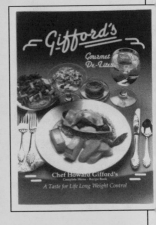

Vitality House is pleased to offer you an exciting work from a professional chef, Howard Gifford, whose meals have astonished guests at weight loss health resorts. Says Howard, "I love to create that which is pleasing both to the eye and the pallate. Preparing healthy food is my medium! My tools? The common everyday household conveniences found in most American homes today. 'Simplicity' is my watchword. Become the creative gourmet cook you have always wanted to be! Learn what the magic of using just the right spices, extracts and natural juices can do for your foods! I'll also give you some helpful hints for shopping and organizing."

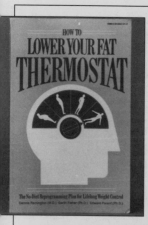

How To Lower Your Fat Thermostat

Diets don't work and you know it! The less you eat, the more your body clings to its fat stores. There is only one program that teaches you to eat to lose weight and it's detailed here in this nationwide best-selling book. All other weight-control programs are based on caloric deprivation. The *How To Lower Your Fat Thermostat* program is based on giving you enough total calories and nutrients to convince the control centers in your brain that regulate fat stores that you don't need to hold onto that fat any more. Then your weight will come down naturally and comfortably, and stay at that lower level permanently.

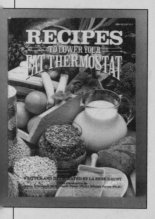

Recipes To Lower Your Fat Thermostat

Companion cookbook to *How To Lower Your Fat Thermostat*. Once you understand the principles of the fat thermostat program, you will want to put them to work in your daily diet. Now you can with this full-color, beautifully illustrated cookbook. New ways to prepare more than 400 of your favorite recipes. Breakfast ideas. Soups and salads. Meats and vegetables. Wok food, potatoes, beans, and breads. Desserts and treats. All designed to please and satisfy while lowering your fat thermostat.

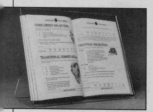

Acrylic Cookbook Holder

This acrylic cookbook holder is the perfect companion to your new cookbook. Designed to hold any cookbook open without breaking the binding, it allows you to read recipes without distortion while protecting pages from splashes and spills.

Desserts to Lower Your Fat Thermostat

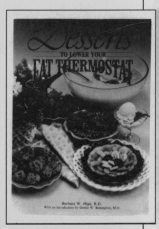

If you think you have to say goodbye to desserts, think again. At last there's a book that lets you have your cake and eat it too. *Desserts to Lower Your Fat Thermostat* is filled with what you thought you could never find: recipes for delicious desserts, snacks, and treats that are low in fat and free of sugar, salt, and artificial sweeteners.

The two hundred delectable ideas packed between the covers of this book meet the guidelines of both the American Heart Association and the American Diabetes Association. They will meet your own tough standards too — especially if you've been longing for winning ideas that will delight your family without destroying their health.

Back To Health: A Comprehensive Medical and Nutritional Yeast-Control Program

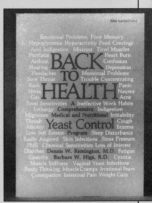

If you suffer from anxiety, depression, memory loss, heartburn or gas . . . if weight control is a constant battle . . . if you are tired, weak and sore all over . . . this book was written for you. While yeast occurs naturally in the body, when out of control it becomes the body's enemy, manifesting itself in dozens of symptoms. Getting yeast back under control can correct many conditions once considered chronic. More than 100 yeast-free recipes, plus special sections on weight control, hypoglycemia and PMS.

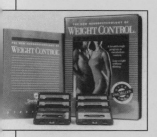

The New Neuropsychology of Weight Control
(8 Audiocassettes and Study Guide)

In the past four years more than a million people have purchased the most powerfully effective weight control program ever developed — *The Neuropsychology of Weight Control* program. Thousands of them have reported dramatic and permanent reductions n their weight.

The New Neuropsychology of Weight Control program is a schientifically-based weight-loss system that teaches you how your body works and shows you exactly what to do to change from a fat-storing to a fat-burning metabolism. Still included are the proven principles from the original program based on the best-selling book *How To Lower Your Fat Thermostat*.

The New Neuropsychology of Weight Control program shows you how to set acheivable weight loss goals and exaxtly what you need to do to reach them. You'll know how much weight you should lose and how long it will take. Included is a complete 12-week eating plan that provides daily menus, meal plans, tasty recipes, cooking instructions and eight shopping lists. You'll know exactly what to cook and how to cook it. And. you'll learn to create your own delicious meals that taste good while helping you to lose weight permanently.

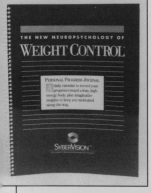

The Neuropsychology of Weight Control
Personal Progress Journal

The journal will be your year-long record of how well you're doing. It also provides information on nutrition, exercise and health.

The Will To Change
(Videocassette)

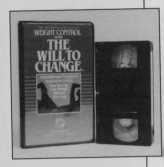

For some people, seeing is believing. While reviewing the key points of the program and the benefits of reaching your goal weight, this motivational video also features testimonials by people who have had dramatic success. In moments of doubt or discouragement, this video provides the needed support and encouragement.

SyberVision's Neuropsychology of Self-Discipline
The Master Key to Success

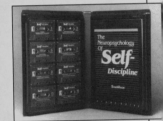

There's one critical characteristic that makes the difference between success and failure; self-discipline. Without it, you can never hope to achieve your ambitions. With it, there's no goal you can't reach.

The Neuropsychology of Self-Discipline is a unique self-improvement program that allows you to instill a new and powerful self-mastery into our own mind and body. Armed with tools, insights, and skills of a highly disciplined achiever, you'll be able, for the first time in your life, to systematically pursue and successfully realize your most important goals.

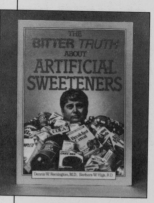

The Bitter Truth About Artificial Sweeteners

Research proves that those people using artificial sweeteners tend to gain more weight. Not only do artificial sweeteners enchance the desire for sweets, they also cause many unpleasant side effects in addition to raising the fat thermostat. Learn the real truth about artificial sweeteners and sugars. Learn how they affect your health and weight and what you can do about them.

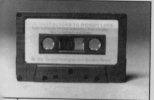

Five Roadblocks to Weight Loss (Audiocassette)

If you have a serious weight problem that has failed to respond to the fat thermostat program, then you could be suffering from any of the five roadblocks to weight loss: food addictions, artificial sweeteners, food allergies, yeast overgrowth, and stress, Learn what these roadblocks are, what to do about them. and how the fat thermostat program relates to them . . . in an exclusive interview with Drs. Dennis Remington and Edward Parent.

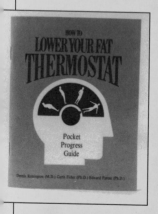

Pocket Progress Guide

A pocket-sized summary of the fat thermostat program that includes food composition tables, daily records, and a progress summary for quick and easy reference and record-keeping anytime, anywhere.

Qty.	Code	Description	Retail	Subtotal
	A	How To Lower Your Fat Thermostat	$9.95	
	B	Recipes To Lower Your Fat Thermostat	$14.95	
	C	Acrylic Cookbook Holder	$9.95	
	D	Neuropsychology of Weight Control (8 Audiocassettes & Study Guide)*	$79.95	
	E	Back To Health	$9.95	
	G	Bitter Truth About Artificial Sweeteners	$9.95	
	H	Five Roadblocks to Weight Loss (Audiocassette)	$7.95	
	I	Pocket Progress Guide	$2.95	
	J	The Will to Change (Videocassette)	$29.95	
	L	Neuropsychology of Self-Discipline (8 Audiocassettes & Study Guide)*	$69.95	
	M	Personal Progress Journal (For Neuropsychology of Weight Control)	$14.95	
	N	Desserts to Lower Your Fat Thermostat	$12.95	
	O	Gifford's Gourmet De-Lites	$12.95	
	P	Easy Gourmet Menus to Lower Your Fat Thermostat †	$13.95	
	S	Gifford's Gourmet De-Lites Spice Mix Set †	$20.95	
Shipping and handling, $2.00 for the first item, $.50 each additional item. (Within the United States).				
Canadian orders add extra $3.00 (U.S. dollars) for 1st item, $2.00 for each additional.				+
Utah residents add 6.25% sales tax.				+
Prices subject to change without notice.			**TOTAL**	

*Purchase code "D" or code "L" and obtain your choice of a FREE book up to $14.95 in value.
 Be sure to indicate which book you would like.
†Purchase code "P" and code "S" together and receive a $5.00 discount.

Ship to: Name——————————————————————

Address——————————————————————

City——————————————— State———— Zip————

Phone (   )———————————————————
☐ Check ☐ Money Order ☐ MasterCard ☐ VISA ☐ American Express

Card No.————————————————— Expires————

Signature ————————————————————————

Mail to: 1675 No. Freedom Blvd. #11-C   Provo, UT 84604   (801) 373-5100
Copyright© 1990 Vitality House International. Orders shipped upon receipt. Allow 2-3 weeks shipping.

To Order: Call Toll Free 1-800-637-0708 or FAX 801-373-5370